I0416981

Essential Oils

Contents

CHAPTER ONE What are Essential Oils?

The way to health is to have an aromatic bath and scented massage every day.' This was the advice given by the famous Greek doctor Hippocrates *(c.460-377* or 359 B.C.), the father of Western medicine. I, for one, cannot think of a more pleasurable way of keeping well.

People of the ancient world knew about the relaxing and protective powers of plant oils; they used them to guard themselves against contagious diseases and infections.

The therapeutic aims and methods of using aromatics have not fundamentally changed since the times of

Hippocrates, but they have expanded and improved.

With today's scientific knowledge we understand more about why essential oils have either antiviral, antifungal or antibacterial properties. The fact that I have been in regular daily contact with essential oils through my work as an aromatologist over the last ten years and have never had so much as a cold, speaks for their protective and health-giving properties.

THE SOURCES OF ESSENTIAL OILS

The pure, fragrant substances extracted from aromatic plants are known as *essential oils.* This does not mean that these oils are essential to the life of the plants from which they originate. Rather the term is used to suggest that the oils contain the healing *essence* of the plants. Unlike the vegetable and macerated oils in which they can be diluted, essential oils are volatile and non-greasy.

Essential oils are contained in the glands, sacs, veins and glandular hairs concentrated in different parts of the plant. For instance, myrtle oil is extracted from the young leaves and twigs of the small myrtle tree. Marjoram comes from the flowering tops of the herb, while spruce comes from the needles of the spruce tree. Ylang ylang is extracted from flowers and cinnamon from leaves or bark.

Citrus oils such as orange, lime and lemon are squeezed from the peel of the fruit, while vetiver is extracted from the root, ginger from the rhizome and black pepper from the seeds.

METHODS OF Application

I work with around one hundred oils which I dilute in vegetable oil and apply in massage treatments. I also bottle oils for home use by my clients. Sometimes I use just one essential oil; at other times I combine two or more oils. I select the oils and the best way to apply them according to the individual client's needs. Oil massage is the most usual form of treatment as the essential oil is quickly absorbed through the skin and is carried by the blood around the body. After six to ten hours it is eliminated from the body (leaving no toxic residue as far as tests have shown) through the urine, faeces, perspiration or simply exhalation.

Professional aromatologists may also give essential oils as intra-muscular injections or internally, mixed with honey water or made into a tablet. Do not use these methods yourself unless you have had professional training.

However, there are many ways in which you can use essential oils therapeutically at home: in baths – including salts, hand and foot baths - compresses, inhalations, ointments, lotions and creams as well as in massage treatment. (See Chapter Seven for details of these methods.)

METHODS OF EXTRACTION

Steam distillation has been the most widely practised way of extracting the oils from the plants since the time of Avicenna (980-1037), a Persian physician who revolutionised the hitherto rudimentary methods of distillation. The advantage of steam distillation is that it lets through only the tiniest molecules, those which make up an essential oil. The larger molecules, including those forming pesticides, fertilisers or other non-volatile chemical compounds, are left behind and therefore do not contaminate the pure essential oil.

The best citrus essential oil is obtained by *cold pressing* or *expression* as steam distillation does not produce oil with the same composition as that present in the fruit itself.

During cold pressing the oil is squeezed out from the oil glands under the surface of the rind. Because the larger molecules from chemical fruit sprays penetrate these glands, they find their way into the extracted oil, so it is important to use untreated crops.

Carbon dioxide extraction and *percolation* are two methods that have been developed relatively recently and, like cold pressing, yield a product which closely resembles the oil as it is contained in the plant. The carbon method involves the use of very expensive equipment while the percolation process seems to be more economical, with promising results.

Solvent extraction produces substances known as absolutes and resinoids, which are, strictly speaking, not considered to be essential oils but the concentrated material from which perfume is made. Jasmine absolute, sandalwood or frankincense resin will contain all the plant molecules soluble in the hydrocarbon or alcohol solvent used in the extraction process. Some of the solvent will also remain in the end product, however. Sensitivity to these solvents is not uncommon and is certainly undesirable.

Solvent extraction is the most ancient method of obtaining aromatic substances. We owe a lot of what we know about essential oils to the methods used to obtain the sweet-smelling pomades which our ancestors wore in order to ward off disease and insects, or the embalming resins used by the Egyptians for their ability to preserve.

But these aromatic compounds are no longer considered suitable for therapeutic use today.

This does not mean that I have not frequently enjoyed giving and receiving a massage or bath scented with jasmine or tuberose absolute. The smell is divine and has a positive psychological effect, just as a synthetic smell can have, but there is little medicinal value in such absolutes compared with that of true essential oils. They offer an aromatic, uplifting experience; not a way of healing.

THE MARKETING OF ESSENTIAL OILS

As a practitioner, I want the natural, unadulterated oil, nothing added or taken away. This is not easy to come by because many growers and dealers have not heard of using essential oils for healthcare. They are used to altering the natural balance of chemical components within the oil to produce a standardised product for the perfume or food industry. Since these are still the biggest markets for essential oils, their requirements control the production.

I have travelled extensively in India to research the use of massage and essential oils in ayurvedic practice - Indian herbal medicine. During my travels I met countless representatives from the perfume and the food and flavourings industry who all insisted that their standardised products were essential oils. They even offered to tailor make them for me!

Sometimes I found the oils were tampered with in the interest of shady commercialism. It is possible to take the cheap and easily available ingredient of one oil and add it to another. The claim of having a pure essential oil can still be made. An added compound can be detected only by an experienced 'nose'.

Fortunately for aroma therapy, an official body, the Aromatherapy Trade Council (for its address, see 'Helpful Addresses' at the end of this book), has become established over the past few years. It carefully monitors the labelling of essential oils, helping to spread better practice among suppliers.

ANALYSING ESSENTIAL OILS

Each essential oil contains a hundred or more natural chemical compounds. The composition of an oil relates directly to its beneficial effects or hazards. This knowledge enables us to choose the oil most likely to help with a particular condition.

Variations in species, as well as changes in growing and climatic conditions can alter the composition of an oil. The chemical make-up is also different in different plants and varies between species and even hybrids of the same species.

The usual way of determining the chemical components of an oil is by using a device known as a *gas liquid chromatograph.* Using this device most good oil suppliers will take a reading for each batch of oil - information that, along with the date of production, is not commonly available to purchasers. However, reputable suppliers can be found easily online.

BUYING ESSENTIAL OILS

If you choose to buy essential oils from a shop, it is best to go to a specialist in natural health products, such as a health-food shop, and not somewhere selling perfumed cosmetics or toiletries. Look for pure essential oils, not blends that are ready mixed in a vegetable 'carrier' oil.

You should buy oils in dark-glass bottles with screw tops and droppers for dispensing. They should be kept for no longer than two years and stored in a cool, dark place out of the reach of children. (See Chapter Nine for further information.)

Ten oils are sufficient for basic and first aid healing at home (see Chapter Six). There is also a wide variety of additional oils which you can add to your collection, although their therapeutic uses are less well established from a scientific perspective. These include oils such as patchouli *(Pogostemon patchouli)* and vetiver *(Vetiveria zizanioidesi)*. There are several varieties of plants such as basil and thyme all of which yield oils with varying properties. This makes them complex for home use.

Since it is still difficult to identify oils of a particular species of, for instance, lavender or eucalyptus from the high street, and nearly impossible to know the exact proportions of the chemicals contained in the bottle you buy, I will give a general guide to the contents of the most commonly available essential oils and their therapeutic methods and uses.

A properly qualified aromatologist should be consulted for the treatment of more serious health complaints.

CHAPTER TWO The History of Healing with Essential Oils

The history of healing with essential oils has often been confused with the history of perfumery or of herbalism. Perfumery is the non-medicinal use of aromatic substances and herbalism is the medicinal use of the whole plant.

Herbalism and perfumery have their roots buried deep in the rituals and customs of ancient civilisations, while aromatherapy, which uses distilled or expressed essential oils therapeutically, is a comparatively recent development.

Indeed essential oils only became available in quantity following advances in distillation methods. The term *aroma therapy* was coined in the early twentieth century.

Over the last few years the word *aromatology* (discussed in more detail at the end of this chapter and in Chapter Ten) has emerged to emphasise further the medicinal and clinical use of the pure aromatic part of the plant: the essential oil. Otherwise the two terms can, to a large extent, be used interchangeably.

ANCIENT TIMES

It is often difficult to know whether references in ancient scriptures to the use of aromatic plants like sandalwood, ginger, myrrh and calamus indicate the essential oil or the plant in its entirety. Even when we find mention of aromatic substances, these would often have been extracted by the use of fats and waxes – as illustrated in the Egyptian paintings of jars filled with aromatic unguents - and would therefore not have been pure.

Herbalism was certainly widespread in Indian, Egyptian, Greek and Roman societies. We can read their works of reference such as *De materia medica* by the first century Roman physician Dioscorides and *The Book of Healing* by the tenth-century Persian Avicenna, referred to in the previous chapter. These texts record the healing properties of plants, not necessarily of individual essential oils.

Before Avicenna - to whom, as we have seen, we also owe the most significant advance in steam distillation - rudimentary forms of distillation did exist, but it was mainly used in order to extract exotic flower waters. The essential oil produced was an almost negligible by-product, as flowers like rose and neroli contain only minute amounts of oil.

THE MIDDLE AGES TO THE EIGHTEENTH CENTURY

Throughout the Middle Ages and on into the seventeenth and eighteenth centuries, the healing power of herbs was recognised and herbalism was practised. Across Europe aromatic plants were cultivated in the gardens of monasteries and stately homes; in the fourteenth century knowledge of the curative properties of herbs was also prevalent among the rural population during the bubonic plague, or Black Death, when herbs were noted for their antiseptic effect. By 1535 Grasse, in southern France, was established as a centre for making perfumes using chemical compounds and essential oils. Perfumes were not just valued as a way of masking unpleasant smells but because of their protective power against disease.

However, the first recorded recognition of the healing potential of distilled essential oils as opposed to herbs and plants in general was made by a Swiss physician and alchemist named Paracelsus (1493-1541). In his work *The Great Surgery Book* he contends that the task of alchemy is not to make gold from base metals but to develop medicines from plants. He saw distillation as the way to produce the *quinta essentia,* the' healing essence' of a plant.

After this we find mention of essential oils in the official pharmacopoeias of the time. Rosemary, cedar wood, juniper, sage and lavender oils were known to the seventeenth-century pharmacists and used mostly for their antiseptic qualities.

Paracelsus was also important for the link he established between essential oils and chemistry. Today a basic understanding of the natural chemical properties of essential oils and their actions is the key to successful healing work.

THE TWENTIETH CENTURY

By the twentieth century chemical science was becoming very popular. In the world of medicine individual plant properties were isolated, or even synthesised, and used as drugs. In aromatherapy we do not separate the individual chemical components of an essential oil, nor do we use a reconstituted oil. Increasingly we try to research the therapeutic value of the hundred or more different chemicals contained in each oil so that we can understand what effect the whole oil may have when used in treatment.

A few scientists, mainly on the continent, began this process earlier this century. The best known was Rene-Maurice Gattefosse because he coined the word *aromatherapy.* He is also the man renowned for badly burning his arm in his laboratory and for the discovery he made as a result. He is said to have plunged his burnt arm in a vat of lavender because it was the only cold liquid he could find quickly. The pain lessened so significantly and the wound healed so quickly, with so little scarring, that he was inspired to find out more about the healing properties of essential oils. Indeed, he and others used essential oils on soldiers wounded in the trenches during the First World War.

Since then, aromatherapy has been widely used for medicinal purposes in France, and some of the most informative books have been written by French practitioners. Among these are Dr Jean Valnet's *The Practice of Aromatherapy* and *Aromatherapie exactement* by Pierre Franchorrune, an aromatologist, and Daniel Penoel, a medical doctor. Dr Penoel, and other practitioners before him, has prescribed essential oils as part of the complementary medicine he practises. I have attended some of Dr Penoel's lectures in which he showed slides demonstrating some startling results, even in cases of advanced cancer.

AROMATHERAPY

In Britain aromatherapy was established in the 1950s through the beauty industry by Marguerite Maury, an Australian. She was interested in the ability of essential oils to penetrate the skin and preserve youth. Her cosmetic use of essential oils was soon extended into the beauty salons where beauticians were trained to give an aroma therapeutic massage for relaxation and skin care.

This type of aromatherapy is now commonly practised in countries such as Australia, America, Canada and throughout Scandinavia. I prefer to call it an *aromatic massage* to avoid any claim to therapy suggested in the word *aromatherapy*.

Beauticians are not qualified to 'treat' any medical condition and they tend to use ready-blended oils. Short courses in aromatherapy rarely equip anyone to mix oils for medicinal use.

AROMATOLOGY

Since the late 1980s a few training schools have begun to teach therapists the basic medical, chemical, physical and botanical science necessary to work therapeutically with essential oils. Such therapists or *aromatologists,* as well as specially trained nurses and midwives, are now working with essential oils in hospitals, hospices and private practices all over the world (see Chapter Ten).

An aromatologist will use only pure, distilled or expressed essential oils based on a scientific understanding, acquired through training, of their properties and effects.

It is important to remember that, before distillation, aromas were extracted mainly by solvents. These are not essential oils but, together with the whole plant, they form the origins of herbalism and perfumery out of which grew aromatherapy. Their history has been summarised here to put the much shorter history of healing with essential oils into context, and also because some of the traditional uses of herbs point the way to many of the benefits that have been validated in the therapeutic use of essential oils today.

CHAPTER THREE - Helping Yourself to Health with Essential Oils

THE PLACE FOR COMPLEMENTARY CARE

Modem orthodox medicine has revolutionised the quality and length of human life in the developed countries of the world. Disease which killed a hundred years ago can now be prevented or cured with vaccinations or drugs. Intricate surgery has saved thousands of lives, while tuberculosis, hepatitis and even pneumonia no longer massacre whole populations the way they did.

There has been a backlash, however. The drugs themselves have produced some serious side-effects which then also need to be treated. Other problems with our modern system of healthcare include the rising costs of equipment and treatment, hospital-bed shortages and the commercial self-interest that promotes research programmes which do not always provide cures.

Rather than eradicating ill-health, technological advances and ailluence have brought new kinds of illness.

In place of dysentery and malnutrition we now have obesity, bowel cancer and coronary heart disease.

As our orthodox healthcare system has increasingly failed people over the last twenty years, there has been a rise in the popularity of natural or complementary medicine. Ten years ago, when I was first starting my practice, almost no one had heard of an aroma therapist.

Now, there may be some misconceptions about exactly what I do, but I do not meet with the same ignorance or scepticism when I introduce myself. Aromatherapy has taken root and spread more in Great Britain than in any other country. By 1992 the Consumers Association reported aromatherapy to be the fifth most popular form of natural medicine practised in the UK.

Sadly, people still come to me and other complementary therapists as the last resort after a round of fruitless visits to conventional doctors and consultants. In frustration or desperation they turn to natural medicine either because they have found no cure for their eczema or arthritis, or whatever it might be, or because they can no longer tolerate the side-effects of the drugs they are prescribed to suppress the symptoms of their disease. Even at this late stage they may find a cure or safe form of relief by using natural products like essential oils. And even if the treatment with essential oils is only palliative, at least there is no risk of drug-induced disease or undesirable side-effects.

TAKING RESPONSIBILITY FOR YOUR HEALTH

Many illnesses and complaints are the result of personal neglect and ignorance. If you can recognise the early signs of conditions such as pre-menstrual tension (PMT), tiredness or sinusitis and know how to relieve them using natural, non-toxic remedies, you can then manage your health and save yourself from more serious illness. Taking responsibility for your health also means following a diet which is low in sugars, fats, refined foods and alcohol, and high in fresh fruit, vegetables, pulses and grains. Try to strike a balance between exercise and rest, especially if you have a sedentary job.

Doctors frequently prescribe antibiotics for people with colds or flu symptoms who want to keep up with the demands of the office or the family. The danger of antibiotics is that they set to work indiscriminately, killing both the beneficial and the unfriendly bacteria and so upsetting the delicate balance of intestinal flora. Ultimately digestive problems or vaginal thrush can result. Antibiotics should be reserved for saving lives, for which they deserve full credit, and not used to treat minor illness, as they can do as much harm as good.

A QUICK FIX

We are a drug-dependent culture, whether it be for stimulants like caffeine, alcohol, cigarettes or chocolate, or for the' quick fix' nature of painkillers and tranquillisers.

We ignore the long-term consequences of our addictions in favour of short-term relief. The more we take drugs, the less effective they become. Our bodies grow to resist them and at the same time feel we need more and more.

Alternative therapists often view pain, high blood pressure or fever as an indicator of underlying problems, which need to be dealt with by natural remedies, not masked with painkillers, blood-thinners, inhalants, antihistamines, antidepressants, diuretics or a cocktail of these. It is worth trying a massage with essential oils to relieve stress and tension before reaching for the sedatives, or, if you suffer from asthma, trying an oil inhalation before continually sniffing Ventolin.

Faced with someone having a heart attack or injured in an accident, I would be among the first to call for an ambulance. There are all sorts of conditions, from broken bones to aneurysms to the acute pain suffered in some terminal illnesses, which need the skills and attention that only orthodox medical care offers. However, there are many conditions which can be treated naturally and benignly. Essential oils are not a guaranteed cure-all but should be the first port of call before taking such drugs as steroids or even aspirin.

The professionalization of healthcare with the use of high-tech equipment and scientific terminology has played a part in creating the passive patient. The miraculous power of drugs to cure hitherto incurable diseases became personified in the doctor. The idea that the doctor could chase away all complaints and the patient need do nothing has not been challenged until recently with the gradual awareness of the limitations of conventional medical practice.

NATURAL SELF-HELP

This is not to suggest that we should play doctors and nurses; merely that through lifestyle management we can try to prevent ill-health and through the use of natural products we can safely take charge of applying first aid and coping with common, minor ailments.

By describing a basic selection of essential oils and their uses, I hope to empower anyone interested in taking responsibility for their own health at this daily, functional level. For any more complicated condition I advise a consultation with a conventional doctor, an aromatologist or any qualified complementary practitioner of your choice.

CHAPTER FOUR Safety with Essential Oils

Essential oils can be harmful when misused, overused or otherwise abused. Like other household products such as bleach, alcohol or matches, they are hazardous if they are not stored and used with care in the recommended quantity.

Most substances are dangerous when used in excess and essential oils are no different, especially when they are taken internally. The worst case I know about the harm done by an essential oil was that of an accidental overdose.

A four-year-old child swallowed 5-8 ml of clove oil *(Syzygium aromaticum),* after which her nervous system was compromised and she lost consciousness. After a worrying twenty-four hours in intensive care, she recovered and later regained full health. The same precautions, such as keeping bottles out of the reach of children, should apply to essential oils as to any other medicines, many of which would have killed the child if she had swallowed them instead of the oil.

SOME SAFETY TIPS

Essential oils are highly concentrated and powerful products. Some basic but important safety measures to remember are:

• keep essential oils out of the reach of children

• buy and store undiluted essential oils in bottles with integral drop dispensers to minimise the risk of overdosing (only one drop at a time will be released)

• never take essential oils internally unless under the advice of a trained practitioner

• never apply essential oils neat to the skin except for lavender *(Lavandula angustifolia)* or tea tree *(Melaleuca alternifolia)* in special circumstances

• never store essential oils near a heat source or allow them to come into contact with an exposed flame, as they are highly inflammable

• never allow essential oils to come into contact with the eyes; if they do, wash out the eyes and seek medical help if the stinging persists

• do not massage the essential oils into any area of the body where there is an infection, inflammation, recent scarring or fracture, or varicose veins; do not massage in cases of fever or high temperature; compresses or other methods of application may be suitable.

SAFE QUANTITIES AND METHODS OF USE

Taking essential oils internally should only ever be done under the professional supervision of an aromatologist.

Ingestion allows the complete and immediate entry of the oil into the body, whereas the amount of oil which can be introduced through the skin or by inhalation is far smaller.

By following the methods of application recommended in this book and by mixing the advised, minimal proportions of 1-3 per cent - around 50 drops in 100 ml of carrier oil - or 6-8 drops in a bath, you will be operating within tried and tested safe limits.

MISINFORMATION

Books and media reports on essential oils published in recent years have dispensed rules and advice on 'hazardous oils' or 'oils never to be used in pregnancy', and so on.

Unnecessary alarm is caused by quoting research data taken out of the context of the small quantities and external methods of application usually used in aromatology.

The reports often fail to specify whether the cited dangers are a result of internal or external usage; they rarely define which species of plant the' culprit' oil comes from and seldom stipulate the quantity of oil necessary to cause observable ill-effects. In addition many studies have been based on animal testing, which cannot provide conclusive evidence for human responses, which are often different.

THE DIFFERENT EFFECTS OF USING HERBAL REMEDIES OR ESSENTIAL OILS

Uncertainty in this area is due to a genuine lack of knowledge about the physiological effects, both good and bad, essential oils can have. Much of our understanding about the therapeutic possibilities of essential oils has been extrapolated from findings about the medicinal properties of entire herbs. There has, therefore, been a tendency to attribute to essential oils the indications and the contraindications listed for herbs.

This is easily done because there is indeed some overlap in the benefits derived from the whole-plant extracts and its aromatics. I can remember strolling in the gardens of several research centres in India and discussing the medicinal applications of many of the plants used in Indian herbalism. I found myself equating these with the therapeutics of essential oils. It was tempting to marvel over the general but often superficial similarities and to overlook the differences.

Herbal extracts do differ chemically from essential oils.

They consist of larger molecules and other chemical structures which are excluded in distillation. They mayor may not contain the aromatic molecules of which the distilled essential oils are exclusively composed. These variables lead to differences in both the benefits and the undesirable effects of using either therapeutically.

In the world of perfumery and herbalism there are many plants noted for their toxicity, most of which do not yield an essential oil. Those that do, like pennyroyal *(Mentha pulegium),* are not commonly available, thereby avoiding any doubt or confusion about toxicity. The ten essential oils described in Chapter Six are the most frequently used and well known.

A WORD OF CAUTION

All this is not to say that essential oils do not have the potential to do harm. Insufficient research has been conducted purely on essential oils and their effects on people. Although we are beginning to recognise both the health-giving and the more problematic properties of individual chemical groups in an essential oil, we still do not know how these change when all the groups within the oil interact.

It is as well to make use of the knowledge we have so far about the components of essential oils and their effects.

Problems are most likely to arise with those oils containing the chemical compounds known as ketones, phenols, aldehydes or furocoumarins (see Chapter Five). These substances may act as sensitizers or cause a sensitivity to the sun, or irritate the skin of some people when certain oils are incorrectly mixed and applied.

CORRECT IDENTIFICATION

All oils should be sold with labels stating the plant and species from which they are distilled and the major chemical components. Oils which are considered to be particularly powerful because of the chemical components present, such as sage *(Salvia officinalis),* hyssop *(Hyssopus officinalis)* and some varieties of thyme (e.g. *Thymus vulgaris* et thujanol-4), should only be bought by trained professionals who can make good use of them within safe limits.

ALLERGIC REACTIONS, INTOLERANCE AND SENSITISATION

It is believed that allergies - which trigger, for example, asthma, eczema and migraines - are due to an enzyme deficiency in the digestive system. If the enzyme responsible for breaking down a particular protein is missing, the protein molecule will enter the bloodstream unmodified and be treated as a foreign body. The allergic reaction is more acute but similar to an intolerant response, whose symptoms typically include headaches, skin complaints, running eyes, nasal congestion and irritable bowel syndrome.

Antigens, which provoke the allergic response and the creation of antibodies, are usually proteins or simple substances which combine with or modify the body's own proteins. The antigen may be a product containing proteins, such as some washing powders. House dust, pollen, and animal hairs are all derived from proteins.

More obvious are the proteins in food, like meat, cheese, milk and mushrooms. Wheatgerm oil (a vegetable oil), for instance, is protein based and best avoided by people suffering from allergies.

As they are not protein based, essential oils will not cause an allergic reaction. However, it is possible to be intolerant or hypersensitive to essential oils, especially those which have been adulterated or mixed with a

solvent. If you think you are intolerant to a specific oil, check that it is a pure, distilled oil as you may well be reacting to the solvent rather than to the oil itself.

People can be intolerant to almost anything, from coffee to perfumes. This seems to be an increasingly frequent phenomenon. It has been suggested that the growing amount of additives, preservatives and colouring in food products, as well as the increasing number of chemicals used in their cultivation, are making people more intolerant.

For those who are hypersensitive it is best first to test a drop of the chosen essential oil on the forearm and see if there is any reaction after eight hours. This is known as a *patch test.*

When a person suddenly becomes intolerant to a substance they have used happily for years, we say they have become *sensitised.* The aldehyde content, for example, in some essential oils makes them *sensitisers.*

Once you are sensitised to an oil, you will normally react to any oil containing the component which caused the sensitisation in the first place. I have seen this reaction suddenly occur with people using a yarrow oil *(Achillea millefolium),* which contains a large amount of aldehydes.

Some oils with a furocoumarin content arenphototoxic. In other words they make the skin more sensitive to sunlight, so it is best not to go on a sunbed or sunbathe for an hour after using them. This group is formed mainly of the citrus oils and a few exceptions like angelica *(Angelica archangelica).* It is wise always to err on the side of caution and follow recommended guidelines when using essential oils for healing at home. But as long as you treat essential oils with the respect they deserve, there is no need to be concerned.

CHAPTER FIVE - Chemistry and Botany

Ionrder to use essential oils safely and effectively it is helpful to have some understanding of what they consist of and the plants from which they originate.

A basic knowledge of the chemistry and botany involved, or just an overview of their importance, can at the very least guard against the indiscriminate and random use of essential oils.

You can cook dinner without being a food scientist, but a little knowledge about food values and groupings can go a long way towards making the meal a nutritionally balanced one. To know the chemical composition of each essential oil is to have a fairly good indication of both its hazardous and helpful effects.

Likewise to be able to classify the plants from which the oils are derived into their botanical families is useful because a pattern emerges whereby certain therapeutic trends are shown to be characteristic of certain plant families.

I will restrict the scientific information to the minimum, just enough to show you how and why the contents of these tiny glass bottles can have the potential to heal, or to harm if misused.

CHEMISTRY

Carbon, hydrogen and oxygen are the building blocks of life and are contained in all essential oils. They combine to form molecular structures that can be grouped into families of chemicals.

CHEMICAL FAMILIES

The main chemical families we will be dealing with are: acids and esters, alcohols, aldehydes, coumarins, esters, ketones, lactones, oxides, phenols and terpenes. The chemical constituents of each family have a characteristic molecular structure and tend to have similar pharmacological effects, whether anti-inflammatory, analgesic, sedative, and so on.

We can now skate through the most common chemical families, learn to recognise some examples of their members by their distinctive suffix - for example, the name of each alcohol will always end, as in *geraniol* or *menthol* - and note their main effects.

Acids and Esters

Organic acids rarely exist on their own in essential oils and only in small amounts. They combine with an alcohol to form esters, which commonly end -*ate*, e.g. *linalyl acetate*.

They are calming and tonic in their effect, anti-inflammatory, antifungal, encourage the formation of scar tissue and reduce muscle spasm. These qualities make them particularly useful for treating skin complaints.

Lavender i*Lavandula angustifolia* and *L. vera)* is the best known example of an essential oil with a high ester content.

Alcohols

These end -*01,* e.g. *eucalyptol* and are stimulating and

strongly bactericidal in their effect. Essential oils which contain alcohols are good for treating children as they are generally non-toxic and do not irritate the skin. You can safely use

German chamomile *(Matricaria chamomilla)* for small children and babies.

Aldehydes

They either end *-al* or have the word *aldehyde* in their name, e.g. *citral* or *cinnamic aldehyde.* Being calming to the nervous system, they are useful hypotensives (i.e. they lower blood pressure). They are cooling as they cause dilation of the veins and are good anti-inflammatories, as well as being antiviral. If used carelessly they can sensitise the skin, causing a rash in some people which will reappear every time an oil containing an aldehyde is used.

Cinnamon bark *i Cinnamomum zeylanicum)* and lemongrass *(Cymbopogon citratus)* both have a high aldehyde content.

Ketones

They usually end *-one,* e.g. *menthone.* There are greater variations in the structure and thus the workings of members of this family compared with other chemical groupings. They are generally sedative, wound healing (by encouraging the formation of scar tissue) and they break down mucus and fat. Some variations have been found to be expectorant, stimulant, analgesic, anti-inflammatory and anticoagulant in their effects.

Ketones are also considered neurotoxic (toxic to the nervous system), although this seems to depend on the precise form of ketone present. For example, there are differences in the structure and therefore the effect of thujone (present in a species of thyme - e.g. *Thymus vulgaris* ct thujanol-4) and carvone (present in caraway - *Carum carvi).* Until more research is done and unless you are an experienced practitioner, it is safest not to use oils containing high amounts of ketones on pregnant women, babies or people suffering from epilepsy. These include sage *(Salvia c?fficinalis)*, hyssop *(Hyssopus c?fficinalis)*and aniseed *(Pimpinella anisum)* as the most commonly available.

Lactones

Because the molecules of this chemical grouping are too large to come through distillation, they are present only in expressed oils - the citrus group. They are cooling, and break down and expel mucus. Coumarins, the largest members of this group, are uplifting in their effect, though they can be sedative and are good hypotensives.

Furocoumarins are known for the photosensitivity they induce. Mter using oils like bergamot *(Citrus bergamia)* or orange *(Citrus aurantiumy,* containing large amounts of these, it is best not to sunbathe or take a sun bed for a couple of hours.

Oxides

Opinion is divided about the difference between oxides and phenols, so they should be approached as cautiously as you would a phenol. Although oxides are rare, 1,8 cineole or eucalyptol is commonly used as it is contained in eucalyptus oil *(Eucalyptus globulus].* Because this oxide efficiently breaks down mucus, it relieves coughs, colds and respiratory congestion. However, it is a skin irritant.

Phenols

Like alcohols these end - *ol.* To avoid any confusion with alcohols, their names simply have to be learnt. The most common ones are *carvacrol, eugenol* and *thymol.* They are very powerful germ-fighting agents, stimulating to both the nervous and the immune system, but can be a skin irritant and toxic to the liver. Essential oils containing phenols should not be overused in either frequency or quantity. For example, clove oil *(Syzygium aromaticum)* relieves specific localised conditions such as toothache but should not be swallowed.

Terpenes

Terpenes, because of their chemical structure, have hardly any aroma but are present in almost all essential oils. They have the ending *-ene* - e.g. *pinene* and *phellandrene* – and are considered to be antiseptic, bactericidal, antiviral, analgesic and stimulating to the immune system. Perhaps their most important action is as quenchers: their presence is thought to dilute or .quench' the more irritant effects of other chemicals in the oil. They do have a small amount of aroma, despite the disregard they receive from the perfumers who often de-rerpenate oils.

Technological advances have made it possible to identify some of the molecules which make up essential oils. But there are still many undetected components within these complex chemical structures and their effects remain unknown. Nevertheless, the essential oil trade is beginning to list those known and researched constituents present in their oils so that users can place them into their chemical families, and have some guide as to their likely pharmacological effect.

CHEMICAL VARIABILITY

Growers and suppliers find it difficult to provide exact information about the quantity of each of the main components contained in an oil. Changes in the soil, the climate and when the crop is harvested mean that no chemical will be present in the same proportions at each distillation.

Controlling the growing conditions can reduce these variations. But since the presence of some constituents can vary from 20-70 per cent, a sample of each distillation should be analysed to determine its contents. Readings can be taken by a gas-liquid chromatography. Traders argue that this is not foolproof as well as being expensive, while consumers increasingly want to know what they are buying.

It must be said, however, that there is no direct and simple connection between the individual constituents of an essential oil and its overall effects. The make-up of an oil is intricate; it is more than the sum of its parts. The different chemicals work together to produce a set of effects which often differ from their individual indications.

These complications also explain why a synthetic oil cannot be a substitute for a true essential oil. An aroma can be reconstituted to make a perfume or a chemical can be isolated to make a drug, but the therapeutic action of an essential oil owes more than we have yet defined to the complex synergy of its chemical components.

Until there has been more research we can only use what has been discovered so far about the chemistry of essential oils as a general guide to their possible effects.

BOTANY

All plants are classified according to their similarities into botanical families. There are around twenty families containing in total some two hundred plants which produce essential oils.

Not all of these are suitable for aromatherapy; some are used only by the food or fragrance industry.

PLANT FAMILIES

The botanical family names are of Latin derivation and end - *aceae,* e.g. *Rutaceae* or *Lauraceae.* Botanical families are plant groups and, just as we would expect members of a human family to have similar physical characteristics, so members of the same plant family share the same structural characteristics. For example, in the Umbelliferae family all the members have the same umbrella-shaped flower heads.

In the same way, the essential oil that comes from each botanical family seems to have connnon physiological effects on people. For example, the Myrtaceae family includes all the eucalypti, such as *Melaleuca alternifolia* (tea tree), *Melaleuca leucadendron* (cajuput) and *Mvrtus communis* (myrtle). The essential oils derived from these plants are all known respiratory decongestants and highly antiinfectious.

The digestive properties of the Umbelliferae family - e.g. *Carum carvi* (caraway), *Angelica archangelica* (angelica) and *Coriandrum sativum* (coriander) - are also well documented.

The following is an alphabetical list of the main families with some examples of the plants they contain.

The therapeutic trends shown by most of the essential oils in each family are also given. As already stated, it is useful to recognise the botanical family to which a plant belongs because the healing characteristics of a family are carried by its family members.

Just as gardeners have to take care to identify a type of plant by using the generic and specific names if they want to grow a particular colour, texture, shape or size of the given plant, when you choose an essential oil you must clarify the botanical family and the plant from which it comes if you want to be sure of its aroma and likely therapeutic actions.

Family	Essential Oil	Indication
Annonaceae	ylang ylang (Cananga odorata)	calming, hypotensive
Burseraceae	Frankincense (Boswellia carteri), myrrh (Commiphora myrrha)	expectorant, wound healing
Compositae	German chamomile (Matricaria chamomilla), marigold (Tagetes minuta)	anti-inflammatory, soothing to the skin and digestive system
Cupressaceae	cypress (Cupressus sempervirens), juniper berry Uuniperus communis)	astringent, diuretic
Geraniaceae	geranium (Pelargonium raveolens)	antiseptic, calming, soothing to the skin
Labiatae	clary sage (Salvia sclarea) European basil (Ocimum basilicum), hyssop (Hyssopusofficinalis), lavender (Lavanduia angustifolia), peppermint (Mentha x	anti-inflammatory, decongestant, stimulating (except lavender), tonic

	piperita), rosemary *(Rosmarinus officinalis),* sage *(Salvia officinalis),* thyme *(Thymusulgaris)*	
Lauraceae	Cinnamon *(Cinnamomum zeylanicum),* rosewood *(Aniba rosaeodora)*	antifungal, antiviral, bactericidal, tonic
Myrtaceae	clove *(Syzygium aromaticum)* , eucalyptus *(Eucalyptus globulus),* myrtle *(Myrtus communis),* niaouli *(Melaleuca viridiflorai,* tea tree *(Melaleuca alternifolia)*	anti -infectious, especially of the respiratory tract, stimulant, tonic
Pinaceae	cedarwood *(Cedrus atlantica),* pine *(Pinus sylvestris)*	anti catarrhal, antiseptic
Piperaceae	black pepper *(Piper nigrum)*	analgesic, anticatarrhal
Rutaceae	bergamot *(Citrus bergamia),* lemon *(Citrus limon),* lime	reducing muscle spasm
Umbel1iferae	aniseed *(Pimpinella anisum),* caraway *(Carum carvi),* coriander *(Coriandrum sativum),* fennel (Foeniculum vulgare)	digestive, uterine stimulant
Zingiberaceae	ginger *(Zingiber officinale)*	anti catarrhal, digestive tonic, warming

GENUS

Each plant family may have several members grouped together. The name of the group, or genus, can be considered like a person's surname - Brown or Smith, etc. Hence *Lavandula* is the botanical 'surname' for the genus to which the different varieties of lavender belong.

SPECIES

In order to differentiate between plants in the same genus we give them the equivalent of a first name, such as *Lavandula angustifolia* for a particular species of lavender.

This identifies the species within the genus.

THE IMPORTANCE OF LATIN NAMES

It is necessary to refer to plants and their oils by their Latin names - to be as specific as possible when identifying a species of oil - in order to be sure of what you are buying. You should be aware that a number of different plants can have the same common name, for example *Anthemis nobilis* and *Matricaria chamomilla* are popularly known as chamomile. On the other hand a single genus may have more than one common name. The *juniperus* can be everything from a Texan or Virginian cedar wood to a savin or a plain juniper.

This is why it is essential not to be content with a bottle simply labelled 'lavender'. Only the Latin generic name with its species and any other divisions can prevent the confusion of one plant with another. If we consider that *Lavandula stoechas* contains up to 70 per cent ketones, which are neurotoxic and should be used with care, while

Lauandula vera is relatively gentle, the importance of being precise about the plant from which the oil originates becomes clear. It is not good enough to say you want lavender without stating precisely which one!

Although many of the bottles of oil sold in the high street are still not labelled with this information, many of the mail-order suppliers are now listing the botanical details of the plants from which their oils are distilled.

MORE SUBDIVISIONS

There are further groupings below the level of species thrown up by such factors as geographical location or cross-fertilisation. These divisions mayor may not be reflected by changes in appearance of the plant, but the chemical composition and the therapeutic effects of the essential oil it yields will definitely vary.

The following is a list of these junior divisions and their abbreviations which you are likely to find on a retail or trade list.

Varieties

A *variety* indicates an important subdivision of a species. Species often have several closely related varieties. The name is usually in Latin and written, for example, *Foeniculum vulgare* var. *dulce* (sweet fennel).

Cultivars

If the variety has evolved through cultivation rather than in the wild, then it is called a *cultivar*. The name is usually not in Latin and often comes from the person who cultivated the particular type. It is written, for instance, *Pinus strobus* 'Nana' (a type of pine).

Chemotypes

These are probably the most relevant to aromatologists. They refer to plants which are visually the same but produce chemically different essential oils. Many plants have several chemotypes which occur naturally. Thyme is a good example, and might be written *Thymus vulgaris* ct linalool. The abbreviation *et* refers to the chemotype, while the alcohol written at the end (in this case linalool) refers to the main chemical constituent present in the chemotype.

Hybrids

These have genetically distinct parents. The parent plants may be different cultivars, varieties, species or genera but are not from different families. The word *hybrida* or an *x* will often appear in the tide, e.g. *Mentha x piperita* (peppermint) .

WHY DO PLANTS PRODUCE ESSENTIAL OILS?

Essential oils are a product of a plant's secondary metabolism, which also produces the larger molecular structures that form tannins, steroids, alkaloids, glycosides, bitters, gums, and so on. None of these are vital to the plant's survival. *Essential oil* is in fact a misnomer; it is not *essential* to the plant's life like the products of primary metabolism. This process is known as photosynthesis.

Here the minerals and water a plant takes from the soil, the carbon dioxide it absorbs from the air and the energy it draws from the sun are turned into glucose, vital for the plant's nourishment and growth.

The exact purpose and function in the plant of the secondary metabolites are not known. They give the plant its flavour and its aroma but there are likely to be several more reasons for their existence. In the case of essential oils some of these may be:

• to ward off bacteria and fungi (they are nature's antiseptics for plants as well as for people)

• to repel insects or other herbivores

• to attract those insects which pollinate plants

• to heal wounds to the plant (as with animals, a plant forms scars)

• to prevent other plants from rooting too close and threatening survival in poor conditions (a plant can exude camphor and 1,8 cineole which reach the soil and make the conditions too unfriendly for other plants to root)

• to limit dehydration by forming a vaporous mist of volatile oil around the plant to lessen the water lost from the leaves when conditions are dry. This is most commonly experienced in pine and eucalyptus forests where the air is heavy with the aroma from the essential oils. The Blue Mountains outside Sydney,

Australia, have earned their name because of this blue haze which hangs in the air above the thousands of eucalypti.

It is worth observing that, although conjectural, many of the justifications for the presence of essential oils in plants are mirrored in the wound-healing, protective, bactericidal and antiseptic uses we are finding for them to safeguard our own health.

However technical, an understanding of the structure and function of plants and the essential oils they contain will illuminate your practice of healing with essential oils.

CHAPTER SIX Healing at Home

In this chapter I shall concentrate on ten versatile essential oils and their indications in helping a wide range of simple and common health complaints.

These are the oils I use most frequently in treatments and those I most recommend for any first aid kit or bathroom medicine cupboard. If you want to extend your collection, consult the table of essential oils (listed by botanical family) and their therapeutic indications in the previous chapter. Please note, however, that a persistent, inexplicable or complicated health problem should not be treated at home without first seeking professional advice.

For safety precautions concerning the mixing, correct quantities, carrier oils, storage and supply, and methods of application please refer to chapters Four, Eight and Nine.

I will specify each of the ten oils by its Latin name.

The common name will appear in brackets but should not be relied upon because only the Latin name will direct you to the exact species I am referring to. It is as well to pay special attention to the different species of rosemary, thyme, eucalyptus, juniper berry, cedar wood and chamomile. In the case of lavender, where several (but not all) species are very similar, I have listed together those which can be considered as a group.

Finally, when an oil is denoted *bactericidal,* this is a general guide to its potential. It does not necessarily mean that it has a broad-spectrum antibacterial action as some antibiotics do. On the contrary, certain essential oils have a specific action on named bacteria.

TEN BASIC ESSENTIAL OILS

CARUM CARVI (CARAWAY)

Plant family

Compositae

Parts used

Seeds

Main constituents

carvacrol, carvene, carvone, limonene

Properties

anticatarrhal, anti-infectious, digestive and stomachic stimulant

Main country of origin

Holland

Cautions

This oil contains only a trace of the phenolic ether anethole, but there is up to 50 per cent carvone, a ketone, present; children and pregnant women would be best advised not to take it.

Indications for Use

This is a good oil for fighting infections of the respiratory and digestive systems. It has also been recommended for treating vertigo.

CITRUS UMON (LEMON)

Plant family

Rutaceae

Part used

peel

Main constituents

caprylic acid, citral, geraniol, linalool, limonene, pinene

Properties

bactericidal, calming, cooling

Main country of origin

southern Europe

Cautions

The high terpene content counteracts the effect of citral, an aldehyde, which could otherwise be a skin irritant or sensitiser; be careful not to buy a de-terpented oil.

Indications for Use

Its antiseptic and cleansing properties make this oil good for soothing insect bites, minor skin conditions, boils, verrucas and warts. Because it is cooling in its effect, it can help reduce fever. It is also indicated for use as a liver tonic.

EUCALYPTUS GLOBULUS (EUCALYPTUS OR BLUE GUM)

Plant family

Myrtaceae

Parts used

leaves /

Main constituents

cineol, eucalyptol, isoborneol,

pinene, terpineol

Properties

antifungal, antiviral, bactericidal, breaks down mucus, cooling, expectorant, lowers blood sugar, parasiticidal, pulmonary/urinary antiseptic

Main countries of origin

Australia, China, Spain

Cautions

Because of the strong aroma and the oxide 1,8 cineole (eucalyptol) present, it should be used with moderation on small children or people with weak chests; it can also be a skin irritant.

Indications for Use

This oil is renowned for its effectiveness against coughs and colds as a decongestant and as a bactericidal. Used as a spray with a 2 per cent eucalyptus oil content, it kills 70 per cent of ambient staphylococci. It has been indicated for use in controlling cystitis, intestinal parasites, diabetes, chronic bronchitis, asthma, pneumonia and tuberculosis. In India I found it was prescribed to reduce fever in cases of typhoid, malaria, scarlet fever and measles.

JUNIPERUS COMMUNIS (JUNIPER BERRY)

Plant family

Cupressaceae

Parts used

berries

Main constituents camphene, campholenic acid, terpineol-4

Properties antirheumatic, astringent, diuretic, soothing and sedative

Main countries of origin Canada, central and southern

Europe, Sweden

Cautions Because of the diuretic effect, it has been suggested that this oil should not be used in the first few months of pregnancy; however, I have never heard of a miscarriage caused by the controlled use of this oil.

Indications for Use

Its astringency makes it good to use on oily skin conditions, e.g. acne. Ulcers and weeping eczema can also respond well. Because it encourages the secretion of uric acids and toxins, it is effective when applied to muscles after sport, or in cases of gout, arthritis and rheumatism. It also stimulates digestive juices and other secretions of enzymes, which makes it known as a tonic to digestion. It helps in cases of depletion or debilitation.

LAVANDULA ANGUSTIFOUA, L. OFFICINAUS, L. VERA

(LAVENDER)

Plant family

Labiatae

Parts used

flowering tops, leaves -0- /

Main constituents

linalool, linalyl acetate

Properties

antifungal, anti-inflammatory, antiseptic, bactericidal, both calming and tonic to the nervous system, reduces scarring

Main countries of origin France, Italy (grown best at high altitude)

Indications for Use

This must be the most frequently used essential oil. A bottle should be kept in every household if only to apply to burns and scalds. Its action is gentle, making it safe to use on people of all ages and in all states of health. Because it is calming and sedative, it is frequently suggested for relieving stress, headaches and insomnia. It promotes the healing and prevents the scarring of wounds. It can soothe and cleanse inflamed and dry skin conditions. It assists in the treatment of leg ulcers. As an antiseptic, it is useful in infectious conditions particularly of the chest or upper respiratory tract.

MATRICARIA CHAMOMIIlA (GERMAN CHAMOMILE)

Compositae

flowers .0-

caprylic acid and monylic acid, chamazulene, lamesene analgesic, anti-inflammatory, lowers fever through bactericidal action, reduces muscle spasm and relieves nervous irritability, especially in children

Main country of origin France

Plant family

Parts used

Main constituents

Properties

Indications for Use

German chamomile essential oil contains a high amount of azulene which is not present in the flowers; it decomposes from a colourless compound during distillation and turns the oil deep blue. It is this which makes German chamorn.ile such a good anti-inflammatory where there is constriction of the veins. It can be used to treat both internal and external inflammatory conditions, e.g. gastritis, colitis, cystitis, eczema, leg ulcers and urticaria (nettle rash).

I have used it successfully in a case of vulvar pruritus and find it most useful to relieve the vomiting which often accompanies gastritis, or the biliousness and regurgitation of acid associated with other digestive disorders. Its analgesic effect makes it good for easing muscular aches and pains, while its ability to reduce muscle spasm makes it excellent for soothing menstrual and stomach cramps. Hay fever, asthma and many allergic reactions are calmed by its influence.

MEIALEUCA ALTERNIFOUA (TEA TREE)

Plant family - Myrtaceae

Parts used - leaves

Main constituents 1,8 cineole, pinene, terpinen-4-o1

Properties antifungal, anti-inflammatory, antiviral, bactericidal, stimulating to the immune system

Main country of origin Australia

Indications for Use

This oil is becoming increasingly popular because of its antiseptic power. It can be applied neat to the skin and is useful in a range of fungal and viral infections, from herpes sores, athlete's foot, ringworm, to thrush. Its antiviral properties make it worth trying with all conditions suspected to be of a viral nature, e.g. post-viral syndrome (or ME).

MENTHA X PIPERITA (PEPPERMINT)

Plant family

Labiatae

Parts used

Leaves

Main constituents menthol, menthone

Properties anti-inflammatory, antiseptic, expectorant, reduces flatulence, nerve stimulant, tonic

Main countries of origin England, France

Cautions Because of its reputedly high levels ofketones, this oil has been contra-indicated in pregnancy; in fact the ketone pulegone, thought to be abortive, is only ever present in a small amount or not at all in this oil. It would be prudent to check the ketone content of the oil before buying it, however; many rectified oils are on the market which have a menthone content in excess of

15-30 per cent. These should be

avoided.

Indications for Use

Peppermint's affinity with the digestive system is becoming well known. The oil can be obtained in tablet form for the relief of irritable bowel syndrome. Indigestion, bad breath and flatulence can be reduced. Its expectorant quality may aid those suffering from asthma and bronchitis. It can relieve migraines, vertigo, sinusitis and headaches, and I have found that it soothes insect bites and sunburn. As a stimulant it comes into its own for combating general fatigue but if overused it can cause insomnia. Jean Valnet suggests its use in cases of scanty or painful menstrual periods.

ROSMARINUS OFFICINAUS (ROSEMARY)

Plant family Labiatae

Parts used flowers, leaves,

Main constituents borneol, camphor, 1,8 cineole, pinene antineuralgic, cerebral as well as general stimulant, hypertensive, intestinal and pulmonary antiseptic

France, Italy, Spain

Many chemotypes of this oil are now available; children and pregnant women should not use the verbenone type as this ketone is neurotoxic.

Properties

Main countries of origin

Cautions

Indications for Use

Being an antiseptic oil, and both a physical and mental stimulant, it is useful for the treatment of fatigue, memory loss, coughs and colds as well as stiff and tired muscles.

Debilitating conditions involving pain and weakness benefit the most, whether it be painful periods or fainting and vertigo.

ZINGIBER OFFICINALE (GINGER)

Plant family

Zingiberaceae

Part used

 rhizome

Main constituents

cineol, citral, d-phellandrene, gingerol, isoborneol, zingiberene

Properties

antiseptic, digestive aid, expels mucus and relieves flatulence

Main countries of origin

China, Philippines, Sri Lanka

Indications for Use

Ginger is useful in cases where there is a loss of appetite and digestive difficulty, such as nausea, flatulence or constipation. It is antiseptic and warming and helps to remove mucus, which makes it a good choice for bronchial complaints. Rheumatic and muscular conditions, where stiffness and cold are a problem, respond well to ginger oil massage.

CASE AILMENTS FOR HEALING AT HOME WITH THE TEN BASIC ESSENTIAL OILS

I offer a telephone advice service for one hour each day to existing clients of my practice. This sets aside time to discuss any urgent developments relating to their treatment and enables me to advise a course of action, often involving essential oils, that they can take at home until our next appointment. It also gives them the opportunity to check how best to use the essential oils (I normally suggest the ten listed in this chapter) they keep at home to treat any other minor ailments or in situations requiring first aid to be applied themselves or their families.

A table follows showing the most common problems and my suggestions for helpful oils to use. For quantities and full details on applications, see Chapter Seven. Since I am restricting my recommendations to the ten basic oils as described in this chapter, I will use their common names but please refer back to their correct Latin tide before trying any of these examples.

On the whole, applying little and often is the best way to achieve results. For example, taking an inhalation of moderate strength three times a day is better than one super-strong one once a day.

It is best to use a combination of all the oils listed for a complaint rather than one individual oil, except for when there is only one oil mentioned.

Complaint	Oils to Use	How to Apply Oils
abscesses	eucalyptus, lavender, tea tree	massage oil, warm compress
athlete's foot	lavender, tea tree	apply neat, drops

		in a bath
bleeding gums	eucalyptus, lavender, lemon	mouth wash
boils	lavender, tea tree	hot compress
bruises	lavender, rosemary	alternate hot and cold compresses
burns	lavender	apply neat to the affected area *Note* first hold the burnt area under a cold tap for 15 minutes or until all the stinging is gone
catarrh	caraway, peppermint, rosemary	diffuser, steam inhalation
cellulite	juniper berry, lavender rosemary	clay application or oil massage
chilblains	ginger, juniper berry, rosemary	massage oil
colds	caraway, eucalyptus, tea tree	diffuser, drops on a tissue, steam inhalation; massage oil applied to sinus area, chest and upper back
cold sores	lavender, lemon, tea tree	apply neat, drops in a bath
constipation	ginger, juniper berry lemon, rosemary	oil massage in a clockwise direction of skin above the colon
coughs	caraway,	massage oil, steam

	eucalyptus, tea tree	inhalation
cramp	German chamomile juniper berry, rosemary	massage oil
cuts and abrasions	lavender, tea tree	bathe affected area and apply oils neat on a gauze dressing
cystitis	juniper berry, lavender tea tree	drops in a bath or sitz bath
dandruff	rosemary, tea tree	add to shampoo or rinsing water
dermatitis	German chamomile lavender, tea tree	massage oil, cream or lotion
eczema	German chamomile, lavender, peppermint (weak dilution)	massage oil, cream or lotion
fatigue	ginger, peppermint, rosemary	drops in a bath or inhaled from a tissue
fleas	lemon, tea tree	apply neat, drops in a bath
fluid retention	juniper berry, rosemary	drops in a bath, massage oil
German measles	German chamomile, lavender, tea tree	drops in a bath
gingivitis	German chamomile, eucalyptus, peppermint	mouth wash
grazes (see cuts and abrasions)		

haemorrhoids	lemon, tea tree	drops in a sitz bath
hangover	juniper berry, rosemary	drops in a bath, massage oil
hay fever	German chamomile, lemon, peppermint	drops in a bath or inhaled from a tissue
headaches	lavender, peppermint, rosemary	drops in a bath, massage oil applied to neck and shoulders
head lice	tea tree	apply neat in shampoo or rinsing water
heartburn	caraway, eucalyptus, peppermint	massage oil applied to abdominal area
heat rash/ bumps	lavender, peppermint	drops in a bath, massage oil, cream or lotion
hiccups	lavender, lemon	inhale drops from a *tissue*
indigestion	German chamomile, ginger, peppermint	massage oil applied to abdominal area
influenza	caraway, eucalyptus, peppermint	drops in a bath, massage oil, steam inhalation
insect bites	German chamomile, lavender, peppermint	apply lavender neat; mix other two oils into a cream or gel
insomnia	lavender	drops in a bath; put several drops on your pillow or add to a room diffuser
laryngitis	lavender, tea tree	gargle

mouth ulcers	lemon, peppermint, tea tree	mouth wash
Muscular aches and pains	ginger, lavender, rosemary	massage oil
nappy rash	German chamomile, lavender, tea tree	massage oil, cream or lotion
nausea	lavender, peppermint	inhale drops from a tissue
nettle rash (urticaria)	German chamomile, lavender	drops in a bath, massage oil, lotion or cream, warm compress
neuralgia	lavender, peppermint	massage oil
ringworm	lemon, tea tree	apply drops mixed in lotion, cream or gel
scalds (see *burns)*		
shingles	lavender, tea tree	drops in a bath, massage lotion
shock	lavender, lemon	inhale drops from a tissue
sinusitis	eucalyptus, peppermint, rosemary	massage oil applied to sinus area of the face, steam inhalation
sore throat (see *laryngitis)*		
sprains	German chamomile, lavender, rosemary	apply in alternate hot and cold compresses

stiffness	ginger, lavender, rosemary	massage oil or gel
sunburn	lavender, peppermint	lotion or cream
thrush	lavender, tea tree	drops in a sitz bath
varicose veins	lavender, rosemary	massage oil or lotion *Note* to avoid pushing blood into the vein, never massage the skin on or below the vein; always between the heart and the vein
verrucas	tea tree	apply neat to the verruca
warts (see *verrucas)*		

CHAPTER SEVEN -Healing Methods

There are many ways in which you can use essential oils at home. As well as using the oils individually, you can mix them together or combine them with carrier oils to create treatments suitable for a wide range of conditions, whether the cause be physiological or

psychological.

Essential oils enter the body by the following routes:

• absorption through the skin in combination with a 'carrier' oil, lotion, cream, gel, clay mix or water

• inhalation through the nose and mouth with air and steam.

The basic essential oils listed in chapters Five and Six are suitable for use according to the methods and in the quantities suggested here. Please see these chapters for the botanical terms and note that Lavandula angustifolia is intended wherever 'lavender' is specified in a recipe.

CARRIERS

Apart from Melaleuca alternifolia (tea tree) and Lavandula officinalis (lavender), which can be applied neat to the skin, all essential oils should first be mixed with or carried by another medium. They are too strong and too concentrated to be used neat.

Air, water, steam, alcohol, an oil, lotion or cream are used to dilute, disperse and then carry the essential oil into the body.

Essential oils can penetrate the skin or enter through any orifice, i.e. nose, mouth, anus or vagina.

SKIN ABSORPTION

We tend to think of our skin as a waterproof, protective coating to keep things out. Many of my clients believe that essential oils can go no further than skin deep until I explain the penetrative ability of the oils. The aromatic molecules making up essential oils are far smaller and more soluble in fatty tissue than those found in most other substances - including vegetable oils, which tend to stay on the surface of the skin - because their molecules are too large to pass through the dermal cells.

Help in clearing up this misconception about skin penetration has actually come from innovations in orthodox medical treatments: the recent advent of hormone replacement therapy, for instance, as well as nicotine patches and the introduction of painkilling gels such as Ibuprofen. These have all helped to spread the acceptance that certain substances can be absorbed through the skin.

As the skin is the largest organ of the body, one advantage of a full body massage with essential oils is that a large surface area is covered, and so a large amount of oil can penetrate. The tiny molecules of an essential oil enter through the hair follicles and sweat glands. Being fat soluble, the oil can also seep through the fatty area between skin cells. The small blood capillaries lying below the top layers of the skin then take the oil to circulate in the bloodstream around the body. Testing exhaled air and urine has shown that essential oils enter the body very quickly after being rubbed into the skin.

INHALATION

The inhalation of essential oils can influence our mood and stimulate memory. It can also evoke a physical response in the same way that the smell of a favourite food can make you salivate. When they are inhaled, the molecules of an essential oil are detected by cells in the nose designed to react to a specific aroma. Since not everyone has all of these receptor cells, there are certain odours which some of us cannot smell. However, a message is sent directly to the brain in response to a smell, whether you are aware of it or not. The part of the brain that analyses the smell is also the part which is responsible for our emotional and memory responses - hence the emotional or physical response to an evocative smell.

After breathing the oils in through the nose or the mouth, a certain amount will permeate the mucus membrane and enter the lungs. This is why oils such as eucalyptus, rosemary and lavender play a valuable part in treating conditions of the upper respiratory tract and chest, such as colds, sinusitis, headaches and some forms of asthma.

The safest methods for healing with essential oils at

home are those which involve entry through the skin or nose. Internal ingestion, whether orally or by using suppositories or pessaries, is more hazardous and should only be carried out under supervision.

METHODS OF APPLICATION *BATHS*

Soaking for ten minutes or so in a bath containing an essential oil offers dual benefits: it will be inhaled through your nose and absorbed through your skin.

Run a warm bath and when it is full add 8 drops in total of up to 4 essential oils of your choice. Halve this number for children and the elderly, halve it again for toddlers, and halve it again for babies. Add the oils once the bath is run and swish the water around to encourage them to disperse. A single droplet could sting you if you sat on it!

Essential oils are not fully soluble in water, so you may want to mix them with a substance containing fat, such as oil or milk. Milk is often the preferred option for a baby's bath. The disadvantage of mixing them with a vegetable oil is that it can leave a greasy ring around your bath. The advantage is that your skin benefits from the softening and moisturising effect of the vegetable oil.

It is now possible to buy bath dispersants for essential oils from some mail-order companies. These are vegetable-derived, natural emulsifiers which, when mixed with essential oils, allow them to disperse fully in water.

Recipe for Relaxation

geranium 2 drops

lavender 4 drops

orange 2 drops

Recipe for Revitalisation

lemon 4 drops

peppermint 2 drops

rosemary 2 drops

Recipe for Soothing Aches and Pains

black pepper 2 drops

juniper berry 2 drops

lavender 2 drops

rosemary 2 drops

CLAY

The minerals and trace elements found in clay mean it is beneficial in its own right. Its astringent and detoxifying properties make it useful for drawing impurities from the skin. In turn the drawing action can stimulate local blood supply and increase the effect of the essential oils mixed with it.

Mix essential oils with clay in the same proportions as for vegetable oils (see under *Massage).* Add them to dry powder and mix with enough floral or spring water to make a paste. Once you obtain the desired consistency, you can apply the paste to the area to be treated and leave it for 10-15 minutes.

Clay packs are commonly used in hair treatments and as face packs for oily skin. Powdered clay for therapeutic purposes is available.

Recipe for Treating Acne

clay 10 mg

bergamot 1 drop

tea tree 1 drop

Recipe for Treating Dry Skin

clay 10 mg

German chamomile 2 drops

Recipe for Treating Oily Skin

clay 10 mg

lavender 1 drop

tea tree 1 drop

COMPRESSES

Compresses can be applied either hot or cold. To prepare a compress, soak a piece of absorbent, cotton cloth in a bowl of boiled and cooled water. To every half-pint of water add 8 drops of the selected oil or combination of oils (see recipes below). Squeeze the cloth and put it on the area of the body to be treated. For hot compresses you can place a hot water bottle on top; for cold compresses you can place a bag of frozen peas or a medical freezer bag on top. Each compress should be left on for 10 minutes. The treatment can be repeated 3-4 times a day, if necessary.

A hot compress is best for treating dull pain or stiffness, while a cold one is good for inflammation, For sprains and bruises, alternate hot and cold compresses using hyssop, lavender and rosemary oils to help reduce the swelling. A compress is useful for treating stomach and head pain, using German chamomile and lavender oils; for boils and insect bites, using peppermint and German chamomile; and some arthritic pain, accompanied by inflammation, responds well to a mixture of juniper berry, lavender and German chamomile.

Recipe for Clearing Head Colds

German chamomile 4 drops

lavender 4 drops

Recipe for Easing Stiff Joints

black pepper 4 drops

German chamomile 4 drops

Recipe for Reducing Inflammation

German chamomile 4 drops

juniper berry 4 drops

Recipe for Treating Boils and Insect Bites

lavender 4 drops

tea tree 4 drops

Recipe for Treating Headaches

eucalyptus 6 drops

peppermint 2 drops

DIFFUSERS AND VAPORISERS

Many of these are now available for use with essential oils.

They range from the simple pottery burner used with a night light to an electrically powered unit. The vapours released after heating contain the chosen essential oil and are diffused into the atmosphere.

Diffusers are a good way of deodorising the atmosphere, for example with pine or lemon oil. Some people with allergies to house dust, *mites* or pollen find the effect of these antiseptic or calming oils released into the atmosphere very helpful. In a sickroom they can have an anti-infectious or bactericidal effect, depending on the oil you choose. In the case of head colds, a decongestant or expectorant oil such as eucalyptus or rosemary discharged into the room throughout the night can offer relief. A sedative oil such as lavender may aid sleep.

Essential oils should be used neat or added to water, depending on the variety of diffuser you are using. They should never be mixed with a vegetable oil in this situation. The number of drops you use depends on how long you want the oil to burn and how large an area you want to cover. Manufacturers of some electric diffusers recommend that you run them for 15 minutes every 2 hours.

Because essential oils are highly flammable, I prefer the electric diffusers. Anything which uses a bare flame like a candle or night light introduces the risk of the oil coming into contact with a direct heat source. For this reason I am also cautious about the use of light-bulb rings which sit around the top of a light bulb. If you do use these, the essential oil should only ever be put in the ring when the bulb is cold and the light switched off.

A cheaper method of creating a room vaporiser is to put a small towel soaked in warm water mixed with some drops of essential oil over a hot radiator. This works beautifully during the winter.

DIRECT INHALATION

One or 2 drops of essential oil on a handkerchief, tissue or pillow, which can be sniffed whenever needed, has a stimulating or calming effect depending on the oil chosen.

While revising for exams, driving a long distance or simply when you are feeling weary, inhalation of an oil such as rosemary is a convenient way to perk yourself up. Equally, using vetiver you can calm yourself in a tense situation, such as before an interview, or use lavender to relax yourself in order to go off to sleep.

HAND AND FOOT BATHS

Fill a bowl with hot water, adding one of the recipes listed below and soaking the hand or foot for 10 minutes 3-4 times a day, depending on the condition being treated. For children, start with only 1 drop of the recipe you are using.

Recipe for Easing Sprains

lavender 3 drops

rosemary 3 drops

Recipe for Reducing Bruising

hyssop 2 drops

lavender 4 drops

Recipe for Soothing Eczema

German chamomile 3 drops

lavender 3 drops

GARGLES

For sore throats, 2-3 drops of a soothing and anti-infectious oil, such as tea tree or lavender, mixed into a glass of water can offer relief and fight infection before it reaches the chest. Before each gargle, stir the water as essential oils are not soluble in water. Repeat twice a day and do not swallow.

JACUZZIS

These offer the best way of using essential oils in a bath. The movement of the water disperses the oils very effectively and reduces the problem of them sitting on the surface of the water and not penetrating the skin.

It is advisable not to use essential oils mixed with a vegetable oil in a jacuzzi as the vegetable oil may clog and damage the pump. (See *Baths* above for recipes.)

MASSAGE

Vegetable Oils

These are the most commonly used *carriers* for applying essential oils to the skin. Mineral oil, which is often used for babies, is not suitable as it does not so easily absorb the essential oils and tends to sit on the skin. There are a variety of vegetable oils, all with their own therapeutic properties (for more details see the next chapter). Always buy cold-pressed vegetable oils because this is the only production method that avoids contamination from any chemical processing.

Vegetable oils are fatty, and because essential oils are fat soluble, they blend well together. Vegetable oils fix or hold the volatile essential oils so that they can soak into the skin.

Once mixed, the oils can be self-applied to a specific area of the body or given in a full or partial body massage.

Vegetable oils are excellent for massage because they give slippage so that the therapist's hands do not drag on the skin.

The proportion of essential oil to vegetable oil is usually 2-3 per cent for adults (halve this quantity for children, and halve it again for babies). Twenty drops of essential oil make roughly 5 ml. The ratio works out at:

• 1 drop of essential oil to every 2 ml of carrier oil

• 5 drops of essential oil to every 10 ml of carrier oil.

Try not to blend more than you need for one application since the mixture will oxidise and lose its therapeutic value. (See the section at the end of this chapter on blending and storing larger amounts.)

The total quantity depends on the area you are going to cover. A full body massage normally takes between 10 and 15 ml of oil, depending on the size and the weight of the person, the dryness of the skin and the amount of body hair.

Recipe for Reducing Stretch Marks

peach kernel oil 8 ml

rose hip oil 2 ml

neroli 5 drops

Recipe for Treating Varicose Veins

sunflower oil 8 ml

St John's Wort oil 2 drops

lavender 2 drops

lemon 3 drops

Note; Do not massage directly over a varicose vein.

Massage can be an excellent way of relieving conditions that have an emotional and psychological aspect:

Recipe for Dispelling Lethargy

sunflower oil 10 ml

juniper berry 2 drops

rosemary 2 drops

Recipe for Relieving Pre-Menstrual Tension (PMT)

almond oil 10 ml

clary sage 1 drop

fennel 2 drops

geranium 1 drop

Recipe for Relieving Stress/Tension

apricot oil 10 ml

lavender 2 drops

ylang ylang 3 drops

Recipe for Treating Depression

almond oil 8 ml

geranium 2 drops

bergamot 3 drops

Recipe for Treating Insomnia

almond oil 8 ml

lime blossom oil 2 drops

bergamot 2 drops

lavender 3 drops

Lotions and Creams

Lotions and creams have the advantage of being less greasy than vegetable oils and often soak more quickly into the skin. Add essential oils in the same proportion as you would for mixing with a vegetable oil (see above).

Natural, non-fragrant lotions and creams suitable for carrying essential oils are available from many online suppliers Some of these can be supplemented by mixing in vegetable oils or floral waters. The most convenient types are manufactured in such a way that you can add essential oils without using heat for blending.

For self-application, lotions and creams are convenient as they rub in easily and do not stain or discolour clothing, as do oil blends. Creams are usually best suited to hand or face treatments.

Recipe for Moisturising Dry Skin

lotion 7 ml

evening primrose oil 3 ml

geranium 5 drops

Recipe for Treating Bruises

lotion 7 ml

arnica oil 3 ml

lavender 3 drops

rosemary 2 drops

Recipe for Treating Cuts and Sores

lotion 7 ml

mullein oil 3 ml

lavender 3 drops

Gels

Gel-based materials derived from natural polysaccharides (do not use petroleum-based gels as these are composed of mineral rather than organic compounds) are less oily than vegetable oils, creams and lotions. This means that they are less slippery and easier to apply, especially for someone with arthritic hands, for instance, where using a cream or oil could be awkward. As with lotions and creams, gels leave no oil stains on clothing. (Like lotions and creams, these are available from mail-order suppliers.)

Recipe for Easing Stiff Joints

gel 10 ml

caraway

lavender

3 drops

3 drops

Recipe for Treating Sinusitis

gel 10 ml

black pepper 1 drop

eucalyptus 1 drop

MOUTH WASHES

Prepare the oils in the same way as for a gargle (see above).

Swill the water around in the mouth and do not swallow.

Mouth washes can be useful for treating bleeding gums, tooth decay and mouth ulcers, and after dental surgery.

For these cases 2-3 drops of either lemon, lavender, eucalyptus or tea tree oil, or a combination of these, can help. This treatment is best carried out after every meal when the teeth have been cleaned.

Recipe for Soothing Toothache

water 150 ml

clove 1 drop

Recipe for Treating Mouth Ulcers

water 150 ml

tea tree 2 drops

SAUNAS

Sitting in dry or wet steam rooms is a wonderful way of clearing the head. Decongestion can be aided by adding 2-3 drops of pine or thyme oil to the water to be ladled over the coals in a sauna.

SHAMPOOS

Essential oils can be added to shampoos to enhance treatments for dandruff and dry or oily hair. Use the same proportions as for vegetable oils (see under *Massage).*

SITZ BATHS

Sitz baths can be used to treat thrush, stitches after childbirth, vaginal itching and haemorrhoids. Only 3-4 drops of tea tree, lavender or lemon (or a combination of these, totalling 4 drops) are necessary in each bath taken 3-4 times a day to alleviate the discomfort, itching or inflammation associated with the above complaints. Tea tree oil will also fight the yeast-like fungus which causes thrush.

Recipe for Aiding Vaginal Healing after Childbirth

lavender 6 drops

Recipe for Controlling Thrush

lavender 3 drops

tea tree 3 drops

Recipe for Soothing Haemorrhoids

lavender 3 drops

lemon 3 drops

STEAM INHALATION

To a bowl containing half a pint of almost boiling water add 3 drops of essential oils. Put a towel over your head and breathe deeply, keeping your eyes shut to avoid any stinging. Continue for 3-5 minutes. Little and often is a good rule to observe when you are using inhalations. It is better to repeat the treatment up to 4 times a day rather than increase the number of drops at each sitting.

Recipe for Relieving Colds

caraway 1 drop

eucalyptus 1 drop

lavender 1 drop

When treating children for colds, make up the mixture in a small bottle and start with only 1 drop for each treatment as the aroma may be too overpowering.

Recipe for Treating Asthmatics

lavender 1 drop

pine 1 drop

All of the oils in both these recipes, plus peppermint, are excellent for treating colds, catarrh, sinusitis, coughs and chest infections. As well as relieving congestion, they fight infection and break down mucus.

TREATING DANDRUFF AND HEAD LICE

A blend of any vegetable oil with rosemary or tea tree essential oils can be applied to the scalp for the treatment of such conditions as dandruff or head lice. Warm 20 ml of vegetable oil, then add 10 drops of rosemary or tea tree oil, or 5 of each. Massage the mixture in for 10 minutes and then leave it on for an hour. During this time a hot towel should be wound around the head as the increase in temperature will help the absorption of the oil. Finally, rub shampoo into the hair and scalp before washing off with warm water and rubbing dry. Repeat every other night for a week, if necessary.

PREPARING AND KEEPING LARGER AMOUNTS OF OIL BLENDS

If you know that you want to repeat a treatment several times, it is easier to mix a larger amount of the oil, lotion or cream. To do this you need to take measures to preserve the blend.

For mixing oils you need a bottle made of dark-brown glass. Such bottles are available from any chemist and come in varying sizes. I will give a recipe for making up a 100 ml bottle of blended oil. This measure can be adjusted as long as the ratios of the ingredients remain the same.

Count in 40-50 drops of your chosen essential oil or oils into the glass bottle. Then add 5-10 per cent (5-10 ml) wheat germ oil - this acts as a natural preservative, prolonging the lifetime of the mix. Finally fill the bottle with your chosen vegetable oil. If you are using a heavy or specialist oil such as avocado or rose hip, it is better to add only 20 ml of this and fill the rest of the bottle with a lighter vegetable oil such as sunflower. Remember to shake the oil mix well before use.

Label the bottle clearly, indicating its contents, its purpose and the date it was mixed. Do not keep it longer than necessary and certainly for no longer than six months.

The same method applies to mixing larger amounts of a lotion or cream. Here it is important to add the vegetable and essential oils gradually, shaking or stirring all the time.

PREPARING AND KEEPING LARGER AMOUNTS OF PURE ESSENTIAL OILS

If you find that a certain mix of pure essential oils is suited for the condition you wish to treat, and that you wish to repeat the treatment several times, you can fill a 10 ml dark-brown bottle with your chosen oils.

For example, if you are using 3 drops of lavender to 3 drops of eucalyptus to 4 drops of lemon to treat a head cold, put 3 ml each of lavender and eucalyptus, together with 4 ml of lemon, into one 10 ml bottle. (Use the rough guide of 20 drops to 1 ml.) The mix is now ready to use each time you need it.

A mixture of true essential oils may be kept in a dark brown bottle with a screw top in a cool place for up to two years.

DOSAGE

In describing the above methods of use, I have recommended a dosage in terms of a number of drops of essential oils. Safety regulations require essential oils to be sold in dripper-top botdes. Since these are not standardised, the size of the drops can vary. Only in France, where drops are normally measured with a calibrated pipette, can quantities be exact. Their drops are roughly half the size of those obtained from bottles sold in the UK and US. It is therefore advisable to choose the lowest dosage suggested in this and other books on the subject.

It must be said, however, that given the small amounts of oil, and the gende methods of application described above, a variation between a drop or two should not cause too much concern.

CHAPTER EIGHT - Using Vegetable and Macerated Oils

There is a whole range of vegetable and infused or macerated herbal oils which you can use in conjunction with essential oils. Previously a vegetable oil was used simply to carry the essential oil into the body.

Now aromatologists are recognising that some of these carrier oils have a therapeutic value in their own right.

They can also complement the healing effect of essential oils: they are not just *carriers*.

VEGETABLE OILS

WHAT ARE VEGETABLE OILS?

Vegetable oils are extracted from nuts, seeds or kernels.

They are known as *fixed* oils because they are not volatile like essential oils. In other words they do not evaporate; they are greasy and leave an oily mark on blotting paper.

Because essential oils are fat soluble, vegetable oils are the ideal medium for mixing with them. They can then penetrate the skin during massage or after any other direct application. A vegetable oil is generally preferred if it is light, not too pungent and cold pressed.

THE COMPONENTS OF VEGETABLE OILS

The precise composition of a vegetable oil varies according to the exact plant and species from which *it* comes. The extraction process *itself* will alter the make-up of the *oil.* Generally vegetable *oils* consist of fatty *acids,* lecithin, esters of glycerol, vitamins and minerals. As with essential oils, the therapeutic application of each oil depends on its contents.

How VEGETABLE OILS ARE PROCESSED

Cold-pressed extraction from organically grown material produces the finest-quality oil for both internal and external use. This process is time consuming and costly, however, and there is only a small specialist market for cold-pressed oils, which further inflates prices.

The food industry usually settles for hot extraction, which can change the nature of an oil. Although this process is more complicated, the yield is greater than that achieved by cold pressing. This kind of processing often includes refining the oil still further to increase its stability, thereby prolonging its shelf life. For example, the fatty acids which are prone to oxidation are removed to prevent rancidity. But vital nutrients such as vitamins are destroyed, making these oils unsuitable for therapeutic treatment.

Despite its name, a low level of heat is used in cold pressing - just enough to help release the oil from the nuts, seeds or kernels. The first oil to be expressed is known as the *virgin* oil. Even if heat is generated naturally from the force involved in squeezing out the oil, it is carefully monitored in order not to exceed a stipulated level.

PURCHASING AND QUALITY CONTROL

Vegetable oils are perishable products and should be bought little and often. The problems inherent in storage and instability in virgin, cold-pressed oils mean that some oils like grapeseed are not easily available in this unrefined form. Since the market for high-grade vegetable oils for use in therapy is growing, there are increasing numbers of online companies who can give advice and sell you oils of a quality to use in healthcare.

Risks to be aware of when you choose a vegetable oil are the vast quantities of oils that are non-food grade _ often contaminated with pesticide residues - and used for making cheap cosmetics. Rendered oils should also be avoided. These are the waste oils collected from restaurants and then further refined. Refined oils are often sold as 'pure', which is legally permissible and sounds promising, but such oils are no good for mixing with essential oils.

THERAPEUTIC INDICATIONS

All vegetable oils can either be taken internally or used externally. Vegetable oils are normally consumed on their own, to obtain the benefits of a particular oil, without the addition of an essential oil. However, taking olive oil for constipation may be complemented by the external application to the abdomen of black pepper *(Piper nigrum)* or ginger oil *(Zingiber officinale)* at a 3 per cent dilution in olive oil.

INTERNAL ACTIVITY

Fats or oils are essential to living matter. The beneficial effects to health from ingesting certain vegetable oils cover a wide spectrum. Evening primrose oil, for instance, has produced some remarkable improvements in cases of eczema, while other vegetable oils are used for their vitamin content. Vegetable oils can be taken by adding them to a salad dressing or swallowed neat from a teaspoon. It is best not to include them in cooking since they are changed by heat, thereby reducing or even removing their beneficial properties.

EXTERNAL ACTIVITY

This is limited to the effect the vegetable oil has on skin cells and tissue since vegetable oils, consisting oflarger molecules than essential oils, do not penetrate the skin.

Vegetable oils can be used to treat a number of skin complaints and the most effective vegetable oil should be chosen for each treatment. For example, evening primrose oil is also indicated for the external treatment of eczema.

Suitable vegetable oils can help in the treatment of varicose veins, bruising, inflamed joints, dry and sensitive skin, allergic conditions and reduction of scarring.

COMBINING VEGETABLE OILS WITH ESSENTIAL OILS FOR EXTERNAL USE

Since some vegetable oils are more specialised than others (rose hip, for instance) and these are often the heavier ones (like avocado, for example), it is therefore best to make up your essential oil mix using only 20 per cent of such a vegetable oil. You can then add a lighter, less specific and less expensive vegetable oil such as sunflower to complete the *mix.*

The severity and type of condition you are treating will also determine the choice and proportions of vegetable and essential oils in the blend. For example, for a viral condition causing acne as the main symptom a blend containing 20 per cent hazelnut oil for the oily skin, 77 per cent sunflower oil and 3 per cent essential oils of tea tree *(Me1aleuca alternifolia)* and lavender *(LAvandula angustifolia)* for their antiviral and soothing properties would be appropriate. Any essential oil will mix with any vegetable oil; the secret is to combine oils which enhance and complement one another's therapeutic action.

THE PROPERTIES AND EFFECTS OF VEGETABLE OILS USED IN AROMATOLOGY

Name

almond, sweet *(Prunus amygdalus dulas)*

Characteristics

mild, fairly viscous massage oil; keeps quite well because of its small amount of vitamin E; can calm irritation caused by eczema

Name

apricot kernel *(Prunus armeniaca)*

Characteristics

light textured, easily absorbed; good general-purpose massage oil

Name

avocado *(Persea americana)*

Characteristics

rich, green oil obtained from fruit pulp, viscous and emollient; good for dry and wrinkled skin, thought to penetrate even the lower layers of skin

Name

evening primrose

(Oenothera biennis)

Characteristics

contains essential fatty acids, such as gamma linoleic acid (GLA), that the body cannot make itself; taken internally, it helps combat arthritis, eczema, high blood pressure, high cholesterol and PMT - high doses are needed to achieve lasting results, e.g. 4 g a day

Name

hazelnut *(Corylus avellana)*

Characteristics

astringent; useful for oily skin or acne

Name

macadamia *(Macadamia integrifolia)*

Characteristics

silky textured; rich and nutritive for mature and sunburnt skins; taken internally, it is said to be a laxative

Name

olive *(Olea europaea)*

Characteristics

viscous and emollient; soothing for inflamed skin, and good for treating bruises and sprains; taken internally, it relieves constipation, and helps prevent high cholesterol and heart disease

Name

peach kernel *(Prunus persica)*

Characteristics

contains vitamin A; prevents dehydration

Name

rose hip *(Rosa canina)*

Characteristics

effective on ageing skin and eczema, burns, scars and wounds

Name

saillower *(Carthamus tindotius)*

Characteristics

not one of the more stable oils, so it can turn rancid easily;
useful for the external treatment of bruises, inflamed joints, and
sprains; taken internally, it is beneficial for bronchial asthma

Name

sesame *(Sesamum indicum)*

Characteristics

fairly stable; good for dry skin and as a sun filter

Name

sunflower *(Helianthus annuus)*

Characteristics

light, not too greasy; good for treating skin diseases and
damage like bruising and ulcers; taken internally, it is good for
treating bronchial asthma

Name

tamanu *(Calophyllum inophyllum)*

Characteristics

analgesic, anti-inflammatory, healing

Name

wheatgerm *(Triticum vulgare)*

high vitamin E content; useful for adding to other oils to increase their stability; heavy but good for treating dry skin; taken internally, it can help with eczema, indigestion, varicose veins and breaking down cholesterol deposits

Note; people with a protein/wheat allergy should be cautious and test a small amount first

MACERATED OR INFUSED OILS

WHAT ARE MACERATED OILS?

Macerated oils are obtained by infusing or *macerating* a herb in a vegetable oil. The herb is chopped up and put into a vat of either almond, sunflower or safflower oil, agitated from time to time and left for a few days in the vat (sealed from the air) at room temperature.

For those plants which do not easily yield their essential oils in steam distillation, this is a way of obtaining aromatics along with other fat-soluble molecules that are also therapeutically beneficial.

ORIGINS

The traditional use of herbal oils obtained by maceration stretches back to the ancient Egyptians and Greeks, with their unguents, salves, ointments and balms. These are basically all herbal oils since they contain the fat-soluble matter, including the aromatic extracts, of plant material.

Their uses are recorded in subsequent pharmacopoeias. By the time of Paracelsus (see Chapter Two) in 1530, there was a switch from maceration to steam distillation.

It is only relatively recently that the practice of combining steam-distilled essential oils with a vegetable carrier' oil has established aromatology as separate from herbalism. However, the recognition that some useful essential oils are being excluded from the aromatologist's repertoire, because they are too difficult or costly to distil, has led to a revival in the use of some macerated oils alongside essential oils.

Any medicinal plant can be combined with a vegetable oil in order to obtain an infused or macerated plant oil. Since aromatologists concentrate on the aromatic part of a plant for healing, it is probably most appropriate for them to limit their use of herbal oils to the maceration of aromatic plant material. The herbal oils with no noted essential oil content, like Echinacea and devil's claw, are best left to the medical herbalists to prescribe, or for the informed lay person to use for use in first aid and treating minor ailments at home.

At present there are a range of macerated oils available from several mail-order companies and health-food shops.

It is also possible to make your own (see below).

HOW MACERATED OILS ARE PRODUCED

Maceration of the plant in the virgin, cold-pressed vegetable oil is best conducted over a long period of time.

Quality-control checks through technical analysis ensure that all the active ingredients are present and not destroyed in the process; nothing is added or taken away. The solvent action of the vegetable oil draws all the fat-soluble molecules (including essential oils) from the plant. The oil is then filtered before bottling.

You can carry out this process simply at home by half filling an air-tight container with chopped plant material.

Add any warmed, cold-pressed vegetable oil with 5 per cent wheat germ oil to increase the storage life. Screw the lid on, stand in a warm place for 2-3 weeks and shake from time to time. Strain the contents through a jelly bag or piece of muslin before bottling. The result is a ready to use massage oil.

It is wisest to use up macerated oils as quickly as possible. They go rancid within a few months.

THE USE OF MACERATED OILS

The macerated oils most commonly used by aromatologists are probably calendula, lime blossom, meadowsweet, melissa and StJohn's wort. The most popular uses have been for treating aches and pains, inflammation and strains. For more details, please refer to the chart below.

QUANTITIES

Aromatologists tend to apply macerated oils externally in a 3-10 per cent blend with a vegetable oil. A small amount of essential oil may also be added to complement further

the mix.

THE PROPERTIES AND EFFECTS OF MACERATED OILS USED IN AROMATOLOGY

Name

arnica (Arnica montana)

Characteristics

used to treat bruising and sprains, chilblains and rheumatic pain; some people can be sensitive to frequent use

Name

calendula *(Calendula officinalis)*

Characteristics

anti-inflammatory and wound healing; good for treating dry eczema, cracked skin and nipples; helps heal skin eruptions and sores, burns and rashes

Name

lime blossom *(Tilia europaea)*

Characteristics soothing to the skin; aids digestion and sleep

Name

meadowsweet *(Spiraea ulmaria)*

Characteristics

sedative; useful for localised pain relief, e.g. sprains and stiffjoints

Name

melissa *(Melissa officinalis)*

Characteristics

useful for treating mature skin and water retention in the legs

Name

mullein (*Vetbascum thapsus)*

Characteristics antiseptic; soothing for neuralgia and rheumatic inflammation; recommended for treating chilblains, haemorrhoids and wounds

Name

St John's Wort *(Hypericum perforatum)*

Characteristics for treating hard bruised skin, ulcers and varicose veins; like an embrocation, it increases blood supply to the injured area; rubbed in or applied in a compress. it can relieve the pain of gout. Lumbago and rheumatic inflammation in joints.

CHAPTER NINE - Buying and Storing Essential Oils

To heal with essential oils you must use the natural. distilled or expressed plant extract. You need to know that careful attention has been given to monitoring the plant during all the stages of its growth through to harvesting. distillation or expression. and storage.

QUALITY CONTROL

In order to be sure of producing good-quality oils it is crucial to start out with the highest-quality plant material.

This will be determined by such factors as methods of cultivation. soil conditions. seasonal variations. positioning. country of origin and the harvesting time and technique.

Since steam distillation. and to a lesser extent cold pressing or expression. can alter the quality of the original plant material. it is also important to have confidence in the methods used. The control of pressure used in expression or of heat in steam distillation. along with the length of time taken. should be considered. Generally speaking. the lower the pressure and the longer the distillation. the better will be the end product. The use of stainless-steel equipment. spring water and fresh. Rather than dried. plant material at the site of picking are all preferable.

I witnessed a quaint example of how *not* to distil an essential oil when I was at a hill station in southern India.

I followed my nose to a home distillery: the air was saturated with eucalyptus as decongesting and as penetrating as an inhalation. A hut made of eucalyptus leaves and branches was almost hidden under dense piles of more dried and curled gum foliage. It crackled underfoot as I waded my way through to the entrance.

Inside, a fire pit had been dug into the mud floor, and blue smoke twirled through a hole in the leaf roof. Over the smouldering fire there was a rusted, metal drum.

Eucalyptus oil was dripping into a chipped tin mug out of a kinked pipe coming from the drum.

I was welcomed by a man and his son who ran the operation together. They gave me the mug of oil to smell.

It nearly blew my head off I would not want to hazard a guess at how many times the foliage was recycled. The local co-operative collects and sells the oil on the open market. It was offered to me as suitable for medical purposes!

ARE OILS DERIVED FROM ORGANICALLY GROWN PLANTS BEST?

Oils described as *organic* mean that the plants they come from have been grown to certified organic standards verified by independent organisations such as the Soil Association. The process, involving tests and inspections, is expensive and the costs are reflected in the higher price asked for these oils.

Just as organically grown fruit and vegetables have more flavour, organic oils can have more 'body'. Although it is desirable to grow plants naturally, without the use of fertilisers and pesticides, it is impossible to keep crops completely free of the atmospheric pollution we suffer today. Acid rain, radioactive and radium contamination are harder to control than the use of pesticides. These factors have to be considered when weighing up the merits of using organic oils against the extra costs involved in producing them.

It is obviously more natural for a plant to take the nitrogen, phosphate and potassium (known as NPK) it requires from the soil rather than be given the chemically produced NPK. Interestingly, the NPK molecules, whether organically derived or chemically produced, are in any case too large to come through the distillation process. What is more, 'organic' is not always synonymous with 'good quality'. Badly distilled or poor-grade plants, whether organically grown or not, will yield an inferior oil.

On the whole, I would be content to buy from producers and suppliers who sought to work as naturally as possible with plants to produce 'whole' oils as close as possible in their composition to the way nature intended them to be.

COPIES

Chemical copies or reconstituted oils may make you feel better because they smell nice, but they can neither reproduce all the chemical properties, in their varying proportions, of the natural plant oil, nor, therefore, replicate the therapeutic effects.

These synthetic or 'nature-identical' oils are all sold under the label of' essential' oils and can confuse the inexperienced buyer. It is only quite recently that a small but growing demand for natural, unadulterated essential oils has come about in response to the increase in their medicinal use. The market is, however, still dominated by the food and flavourings industries where the need for uniformity is greater than the need for authenticity.

GRADING ESSENTIAL OILS

When essential oils are rectified or adjusted to a common standard, this is frequently done by adding or deleting certain chemical constituents, making them conform to the quantities present in a previous batch. The oils are the grouped as Commercial, Pharmaceutical, Industrial, Natural, etc., each with its own grade. For example, lower-grade, Commercial' ylang ylang is intended for the bottom end of the toiletry market. The problem is that someone could be tempted by the lower price and misled into buying such an oil for therapeutic purposes.

There are also unscrupulous dealers who dilute or alter essential oils and sell them to unsuspecting people for use in aromatherapy. They might dilute an essential oil with a vegetable 'carrier' oil, or remove a cheaper component from one oil and add it or a synthetic one to a more expensive oil to make up the quantity. These are still sold as pure essential oils!

It is easy to recognise an essential oil which has been mixed with a vegetable 'carrier' because it will leave a greasy mark on blotting paper. However, it is difficult to tell whether more camphor or some other ingredient has been used to make up an oil unless you have a very educated nose. With time and practice in smelling different oils you can begin to discern the fakes as they often smell artificial - too pungently of the raw material.

WHERE TO BUY

It is best to buy essential oils for therapeutic use from a recognised healthcare supplier such as a health-food shop, or an online firm specialising in this area.

It is advisable to steer clear of those outlets which mix health and beauty care because it is often difficult to tell whether the products have been selected with medicinal or cosmetic use in mind. I know of retailers who claim their brand of toiletry can help clear dandruff or acne but the oils the products contain are the reconstituted ones used by the company's perfume department.

Essential oils sold in transparent glass bottles on market stalls and with no verifiable product information but a tempting price are best resisted. I have had countless clients report skin irritations or feeling nauseous as a result of using such products.

WHAT TO BUY

The following is a list of points to consider when you are purchasing pure, natural, distilled or expressed plant oils.

• Dark-glass bottles with integral droppers and screw tops are a good starting point.

• Botanical names are important when selecting the oil you want to buy. They will accurately define the species and even the variety of plant from which the sell-by dates are not normally marked on bottles of essential oils. Without these, or at least a bottling date, it is impossible to know how long an oil has been kept in a producer's or supplier's stocks. Try to buy from companies who will guarantee that they only sell oils produced from the current year's harvest.

• The price should reflect the current availability and demand. Essential oils differ widely in price because the yield varies from plant to plant and from harvest to harvest.

• The aroma of an oil should be dynamic, with depth and vigour. It should not smell too artificially of the plant from which it originates. Not all essential oils smell pleasant.

STORAGE

Because they deteriorate in sunlight, you should buy essential oils in dark-glass bottles. Deterioration happens faster at the blue end of the spectrum than the red, so black or brown glass is better than blue. It is also advisable to store these bottles in a dark cupboard away from direct sunlight.

Essential oils are volatile so a screw top should always be securely tightened. If the bottle was left open, the oil would eventually evaporate or enough of the lighter molecules would be released and what was left would have a different composition.

Essential oils are powerful and concentrated substances not to be used in large quantities. Integral droppers inserted in all bottles containing essential oils will help prevent overuse. They also limit spillage, which is useful because the chemicals in the oils can damage plastic, painted or varnished surfaces. oil originates. The common name may be given but they can be confusing especially in the case of lavender, rosemary, marjoram and chamomile. You should be guided by the Latin name in order to know exactly what you are getting.

• The key chemical constituents should be given for each oil in order to allow you to determine its likely characteristics. At the very least, the listing of these components can make you more aware of how one species of lavender is different from another.

• Cautionary labels are used by some companies who wish to flag certain oils as hazardous. It should be remembered that all oils should be treated with care and what is thought hazardous in one country may be deemed safe in another.

A warm place such as over a radiator is not suitable for storing an essential oil. If the bottle is partly used, the oxygen in the air space can react with the remaining oil.

Oils which are stored in filled and airtight, amber bottles in a dark, cool place will keep the longest.

Although there are reports of oils lasting for years, it is safest to count on a life of two years for essential oils if kept in these optimum conditions.

Oils with a high aldehyde content, such as those in the citrus group, do not have such a long life. The aldehydes quickly turn to acids so that the oil takes on an acidic smell.

When essential oils are mixed with a lotion, cream or vegetable oil, their shelf life is only as long as that of the product they have been mixed with. For example, a vegetable oil with no preservatives will go rancid after around six months.

CHAPTER TEN - Essential Oilsin Healthcare Settings

ALL IN A MASSAGE?

Many people assume that an aromatherapy treatment means a massage using essential oils. I prefer to call this an *aromatic massage.* Massage is a discipline in its own right to which fragrances may be added to heighten the sensuous and relaxing experience.

In India, where I observed many ayurvedic (herbal) treatments, I discovered that massage could mean an application to the skin of any form of herbal oil. Dermal penetration of the ayurvedic preparations, which include some essential oils, is carried out by using hot rice poultices containing oils or by a vigorous rub-down with ladles of warm vegetable oil containing herbs and aromatics. The benefits obtained by absorbing the herbs are of primary importance, while the massage itself is only a vehicle with little value attached to what it may contribute in its own right.

MASSAGE IN AROMATOLOGY

The Frenchman Rene-Maurice Gartefosse, who coined the term *aromatherapy,* did not envisage the use of or necessarily include massage in his work. *Aromatology,* together with *phytotherapy* (herbal medicine), is practised in France today by medical doctors with a specialism in complementary medicine. It is considered a branch of medicine. The use of essential oils is favoured for fighting infections, especially those of the respiratory tract. The methods of application include inhalations, compresses, internal dosage - either oral or through suppositories and pessaries - baths and a limited amount of massage.

MASSAGE IN AROMATHERAPY

In the US, Canada, Australia, Great Britain, the Republic of Ireland, South Africa, Israel and some European countries essential oils are mainly used to restore and maintain mental, physical and emotional health by trained non-medical practitioners or interested medical staff, such as nurses or midwives. These people commonly refer to themselves as *aromatherapists* and use massage as their main way of healing with essential oils.

Training standards, the degree of medical knowledge and scientific understanding of essential oils vary between and within these countries. International Federation of Aroma therapists encourage the therapeutic application of essential oils mainly through massage and not necessarily by qualified doctors. They have introduced courses and schemes designed to establish this practice in healthcare settings such as hospitals and hospices. Although the practice of aromatherapy in these contexts has been growing since the late 1980s in Britain, it is in varying stages of infancy in other English-speaking countries.

In the early days - the 1960s onwards - and even in some countries today, a rather superficial training in the theory of essential oils went hand in glove with a qualification in massage. Even when I started in the mid- 1980s, evidence of my diploma in physiology, anatomy and remedial massage was a prerequisite to my study of and future work with essential oils. Doubtless this heavy bias towards massage as the dominant method of applying essential oils came about because of the cosmetic use beauticians made of oils in facials and body massage in their salons from the 1960s up to and including the present day.

Massage and essential oils certainly form a convenient partnership because essential oils are soluble in the fatty vegetable oil which is used to give the slippage necessary for massage. It was soon found that the fat-soluble essential oils penetrated the skin and entered the blood stream quickly and efficiently when blended and applied this way.

Another reason for the match is that most illness is bound up with experiencing pain and stress. Massage reduces both of these states, while painkilling and sedative oils provide further relief.

Massage has had the advantage of opening the door in some hospitals and various clinics to the use of essential

oils. In the US, for example, doctors were willing to consider the benefits of massage for their patients and tolerated the introduction of essential oils by nurse massage therapists providing the oils would do no harm. The good they might do was initially not even considered.

In many countries, however, the role of massage as the primary method of application for essential oils anchors their use to the health, fitness and beauty centres, and only just allows them to float at the periphery of medical settings.

INCREASING ACCEPTANCE OF ESSENTIAL OILS BY ORTHODOX MEDICAL PRACTITIONERS

More recently, as the therapeutic value of essential oils has gained scientific recognition, there has been an increase in the number of health professionals qualified in other areas such as paramedics or acupuncturists - and in the number of new students interested in learning about healing with essential oils. They do not always want to train in massage, and this is supported by the rising number of clients who do not primarily seek a massage.

Many more now consult me about specific medical conditions, wanting to be advised on what oils to take and how to apply them at home.

In Britain, by the end of 1992, doctors were allowed to refer patients under the National Health Service to any complementary therapist, providing they remained in charge of the case. Doctors and health authorities are beginning to recognise the therapeutic and financial benefits of aromatology. In the US, where there is no National Health Service, private health insurance does not pay for complementary therapies but there is a growing acceptance of the part complementary medicine can play. In other countries like Australia, Ireland and South Africa the use of essential oils in healthcare settings is permitted but often only when the service is offered on a voluntary basis.

This is still a far cry from the use doctors make of essential oils in France, where there is a plethora of pharmacies and analytical laboratories involved in aromatology. A French doctor will have essential oils tested against a sample of bacteria or fungi taken from a patient and order a prescription to be made according to the results of these *aromatograms*.

Although it may be thought restrictive that only qualified medical or recognised health practitioners can offer any complementary therapy such as aromatology in countries such as France or Switzerland, the status conferred on essential oils by the use made of them by doctors acknowledges their therapeutic worth.

Worldwide, steps are being taken to broaden the clinical use of essential oils. This trend and the new, more medical approach have encouraged the move away from the term *aroma therapy* towards a new name that reflects *healing* rather than simply *massaging* with essential oils.

Aromatology embodies this new direction. It neatly avoids the complications implied by the word *therapy* for the Europeans, and the confusion with *aromatic massage* for everyone else.

CHAPTER ELEVEN - Professional Treatment with Essential Oils

WHO BENEFITS FROM TREATMENT?

Anyone can benefit from using essential oils. You don't have to be ill - time spent maintaining health and preventing disease is never wasted. You have a choice between seeking a consultation for guidance about the selection of essential oils to suit your present condition and methods of home application, or having them applied in massage.

I am commonly asked to help with sinusitis, anteand postnatal care, eczema, asthma, depression, anxiety, insomnia, muscular strain and pain, fungal and viral infections, PMT, arthritis, ME and irritable bowel syndrome. I prescribe the oils and the best method of application.

I am also asked to give aromatic massage to people who are in need of relaxation and pampering. In this case I am using my skills as a masseuse and choosing a safe oil whose smell is liked by the client rather than drawing on my knowledge as an aromatologist.

WHAT HAPPENS IN A TYPICAL TREATMENT?

The aromatologist will begin with a consultation lasting from between thirty minutes to one hour, depending on the complexity of your case. You will be asked questions about your medical history, general health and lifestyle.

The practitioner should understand the structural make-up, function and diseases of the body, and may wish to contact your GP or any other therapist you are seeing, with your permission, in order to keep all parties informed about any ongoing treatment.

An aromatologist is unlikely to focus merely on the symptoms of illness or imbalance; the underlying causes will be addressed. This may result in recommendations on changes in lifestyle, diet and exercise. For example, in the case of gallstones an attempt may be made to dissolve the stones using oils, or the patient may opt for surgery. In either event the aromatologist will also advise dietary management and the application of essential oils to help the body's conversion of fats or formation of bile.

Many aromatologists may also have a training in other disciplines such as nutrition, herbalism or acupuncture, all of which may well help in the treatment of particular conditions.

The holistic approach of most complementary medical practitioners means that they will piece together symptoms like a jigsaw puzzle until they get a whole picture of the person seeking treatment. Orthodox medicine attributes illness to exposure to some pathological organism (germ) or to some isolated malfunction in an otherwise healthy body. It then gears its treatment to the specified offender or faulty part.

The aromatologist, on the other hand, steers a middle course, seeing the client as a dynamic whole and the disease as the result of a breakdown in health.

Therefore as well as homing in on the disease itself (such as the application of a bactericidal oil to combat repeated gastro-enteritis), the chosen oil would also be a stimulant to the immune system or a tonic to the liver, the kidney or whichever organ is considered to be weakening.

After selecting and blending appropriate oils, the aromatologist will suggest the best method of application.

This may be through a massage to a part or to the whole body on one or more occasions. It may also be agreed that the client should use the oils at home in compresses or inhalations.

Sessions will usually last an hour. If massage or any other application with essential oils is to be given, it may happen at the same or a separate time.

After a massage with selected and mixed oils, most people immediately experience a greater sense of wellbeing or relief from pain or discomfort. I notice that within ten minutes the oils begin to be absorbed and the person visibly relaxes as they take effect.

In some rare cases it is possible to feel very fatigued or develop a headache after a session. This is normally when people are debilitated, run-down or full of toxins, as treatment can release toxins from the tissues and produce reactions like headaches or diarrhoea. In addition the oils can slow down a person fighting exhaustion but unable to let go. The answer is to pitch the treatment to a tolerable but effective level, and to administer a series of treatments at four-day intervals.

Following an aromatologist's advice to carry out physical exercises, give up smoking or exclude aggravating foods will play an important part in restoring good health.

Attending future appointments and using essential oils in lotions, inhalations or baths at home are suggestions which the practitioner can make but only the client can decide whether to carry out.

It is the practitioner's responsibility to refer the client elsewhere if it is felt that she or he is not skilled or specialised enough to achieve the best results.

HOW TO FIND A QUALIFIED AROMATOLOGIST

An excellent way to find an aromatologist is by word of mouth. But most countries have a lead representative body. By contacting the lead body in your country, you can obtain a list of its member associations and training establishments. There will be a minimum training requirement for members belonging to these bodies: the therapists on their register must have reached a specified standard.

There are some international organisations based in Britain that have branches in several English-speaking countries - such as the International Federation of Aromatherapists, which also operates in Australia. Groups are being set up all the time, and New Zealand is particularly well served with its extremely active New Zealand Register of Holistic Aromatherapists.

Most governing bodies are composed of both aromatherapy associations and training schools. They therefore both unify the profession and establish common standards of training and professional conduct.

In addition they act as a public watchdog and support research in the field. Through close links with other complementary medical groups such as the British

Complementary Medicine Association or the National Federation for Specialty Nursing Organisations in the US, aromatherapy organisations seek to integrate their practice in the structure of their nation's healthcare system.

QUESTIONS TO ASK

You may find that not all professionals are using the tide *aromatologist,* so it would be as well to clarify whether the practitioner uses methods other than massage and what exams he or she has taken in the medical sciences, other complementary therapies and in the theory (including biochemistry) of essential oils.

A good indicator is to ask what length of training a practitioner has undergone. Weekend courses or adult education classes designed to guide people in the use of essential oils at home within the family have been considered sufficient by some to set themselves up as practitioners. Completion of a two-year, part-time course indicates a good level of training, together with the acquisition of other skills in orthodox or complementary medicine.

Association members are obliged to hold insurance for treating the general public and for mixing and applying essential oils. If you do not choose an aromatherapist or aromatologist through the associations, it would be as well to check they have insurance, such as via another professional body through whom they have gained other, recognised qualifications.

A good practitioner will welcome the following key questions:

• How long did you train?

• To what professional body do you belong?

• What examinations have you taken and passed?

• Are you insured?

• Are you qualified to practise any other therapies?

I am always amazed by the number of people who come to my practice and do not ask any of these questions. I offer the information anyway.

CHAPTER TWELVE - Case Studies

The case studies in this chapter are all genuine, although the names have been altered.

CASE ONE - SYLVIA

BACKGROUND

Sylvia's son telephoned me to ask whether I would see his seventy-year-old mother, whom he was very worried about because she had not slept for several days. Her doctor, whom she had relied on for years, had retired from the local practice. He had been prescribing Mogadon (a sleeping tablet) and, with his departure from the practice, the tablets had suddenly stopped working.

When Sylvia came to see me the next day, she was very jumpy and over-exhausted from lack of sleep. She described herself as generally anxious and fearful of illness striking herself or others. Five days previously she had received some worrying news about a friend's health, which coincided with her own doctor leaving. She took two Mogadon tablets that night, followed by another two some hours later. They had no effect. Trying a second night, swallowing Mogadon to no avail, she decided to give them up altogether. The three following nights, in which she took no sleeping tablets, still brought no sleep.

TREATMENT

Her new doctor had prescribed Dothiepin (an antidepressant), which she had taken the previous night.

I explained that it was unlikely that these tablets would take immediate effect and remained non-judgmental about this course of action. At this stage I felt the most important task was to reduce her anxiety and allay her fears about the consequences of her insomnia.

Upon further questioning and physical examination I found that she was in remarkably good health. I advised against taking either caffeine or alcohol in the evenings and recommended a herbal tea containing valerian and chamomile. I finished with a 20-minute back massage using *Lavandula angustifolia* (lavender) and *Ocimum basilicum* (European basil).

In many hospital wards lavender oil has been used in diffusers very successfully in place of medication to induce sleep. I chose the basil because it is helpful with nervous insomnia and debility. It is also indicated for muscle cramps and gastric spasms, both of which were bothering Sylvia.

OUTCOME

Over the next two weeks I repeated this massage treatment four times, taking an hour for each session. Sylvia slowly began to relax and reported an average of five hours' sleep each night. She was experiencing light-headedness, palpitations and drowsiness during the day because of the antidepressants. With her doctor's knowledge, she decided to reduce the dose gradually with a view to stopping them altogether.

Over the next few weeks there was a steady improvement in Sylvia's sleep pattern. I reduced the treatment sessions but gave Sylvia a bottle of *Lavandula angustifolia* to use in a bath before going to bed and to add to a diffuser in her bedroom. She is now sleeping for around six hours a night and is no longer dependent on sleeping tablets.

(See Chapter Three for the discussion about deciding whether to consult an orthodox or complementary medical practitioner.)

CASE TWO - JAMES

BACKGROUND

A local physiotherapist referred James to me to see whether I could help with the onset of arthritis associated with the Crohn's disease he had had for the last two years. James was twenty-eight years old and just regaining his strength following a colostomy performed two months ago, in which most of his bowel had been removed. I found that he was weak with a lot of inflammation in his lower limbs, and had severe back pain. I decided on the oils I wanted to use but knew the poor mineral and vitamin absorption which accompanies Crohn's disease, together with the strong medication used, would make James hypersensitive.

I have found anyone convalescing from a serious illness involving heavy medication and/or a breakdown in their immune defence system, such as in the case of HIV-positive patients, is likely to be intolerant to many substances, including essential oils. These therefore must be diluted and mixed with care.

TREATMENT

I took a skin patch test for *Achillea millefolium* (yarrow) and found that James developed an itchy rash almost immediately.

I then tried *Matricaria chamomilla* (German chamomile) and other oils from the Compositae family - the family to which both yarrow and chamomile belong. It was clear from the negative reaction that I was only going to be able to use these oils at a 1 per cent dilution in sunflower oil.

Mentha x piperita (peppermint) is another possible skin irritant, but I wanted to use it for its anti-inflammatory effect. James unfortunately complained of an itching sensation after using a very small amount in a back massage. I rubbed generous quantities of a plain vegetable oil over the irritated area then wiped away the excess to relieve the sensation. There was neither a rash nor redness but I decided to find an alternative oil.

I chose *Cinnamomum zeylanicum* (cinnamon bark), which has a high content of cinnamic aldehyde - aldehydes are a good anti-inflammatory but are known to be potential skin sensitisers. However, by carefully blending this oil with *Citrus sinensis* (sweet orange), I was able to quench' the aldehyde with the large amount of terpene present in the orange oil. Sweet orange is also a useful digestive.

OUTCOME

I found that, in each weekly twenty-minute session, by alternating and combining several oils while limiting the overall use of these oils, I achieved good results. Through this careful management and blending of oils, beneficial treatment proceeded without causing any unpleasant or uncomfortable reactions.

(See Chapter Four for information about intolerant reactions to certain essential oils.)

CASE THREE - SUSIE

BACKGROUND

Susie, a 22-year-old receptionist, came to see me about her eczema which had developed during puberty. Odd patches had appeared on her legs and arms as a child but now large areas of her back, her hands, her knee and elbow joints and her face were affected. She had stopped oral contraception two months ago and experienced a flare-up ever since.

Her periods had been irregular before taking the Pill and she hadn't had one at all since stopping. She complained that she felt she looked very old and that she even felt stiff, which she found disturbing given her age.

I explained that the continual use of cortisone cream inevitably ages and thins the skin. I suspected that the reaction to stopping the Pill would be particularly severe until hormonal activity settled down again.

TREATMENT

I made a cream containing 10 per cent evening primrose oil, 2 per cent *Matricaria chamomilla* (German chamomile) and 2 per cent *Lavandula angustifolia* (lavender) for her to use at home.

I also advised the exclusion of all wheat, dairy and alcoholic products from her diet. This meant Susie would have to devise meal plans because she was used to picking up take-away food and sweet snacks. In addition, she agreed to drink as much water as she could in a day.

I advised that she took two 1,000 mg capsules of evening primrose oil morning and evening, and one teaspoon of macadamia nut oil a day (for constipation).

Susie came for weekly treatments in which I used cool compresses of *Hyssopus officinalis (hyssop),juniperus communis* (juniper berry) and *Salvia sclarea* (clary sage) on the affected areas of skin.

After four sessions her skin was less inflamed and some areas had cleared enough to start massage treatment with a 5 per cent dilution of evening primrose oil and 5 per cent rose hip oil in almond oil containing *Mentha x piperita* (peppermint) and *Hyssopus officinalis.* I have found that although large quantities of peppermint oil can irritate the skin, small amounts can relieve the itching and inflammation which accompanies eczema.

OUTCOME

Within six weeks Susie had her first period since stopping the Pill. We then timed our sessions to fall once a month before her period was due. Over the next six months her periods became regular, her skin was clear other than when she had a dietary lapse and it quickly resolved itself if she applied the cream. Both the constipation and the stiffness disappeared with the course of massage treatment and dietary changes.

CASE FOUR - PETER

BACKGROUND

Peter had suffered from acne on his upper back and face since he was sixteen years old. He was now twenty and in the middle of a course of Roacutain, an oral treatment for acne based on vitamin A. The acne had cleared but the sideeffects of chapped lips and very dry skin were making him uncomfortable. He was concerned that I should not use an oil that would encourage his skin to become oily again, but he did want to have something to relieve the taut, dry cracking.

TREATMENT

I mixed a 3 per cent dilution of *Melaleuca alternifolia* (tea tree) with hazelnut oil and gave it to Peter to add to his bath or apply neat, whichever method he felt most comfortable with.

OUTCOME

Peter continued with this treatment for six months as his skin was very dry, but over this period it improved greatly.

Whenever his acne returns and he has to take another course of Roacutain, he comes back to me to replenish his supply of oils.

(For cases Three and Four, see Chapter Eight for information about combining vegetable oils with essential oils.)

CASE FIVE - CHARLES

BACKGROUND

Charles was fifty-five years old when he came to see me about his red and inflamed face, the skin often chapped and flaking. He knew he was intolerant to something in the atmosphere or in his diet, but he had never isolated what it might be. Although he had a desk-bound job as a civil servant, he spent all his free time either walking or gardening. Apart from prominent varicose veins and the fact that he bruised very easily, he had no other health complaints except for a permanent feeling of congestion in his sinuses.

Charles felt he did not want to undergo any more tests or trials to identify the allergen or whatever caused his sensitivity. He had a very healthy diet containing no dairy products because he had discovered they increased the congestion in his sinuses. He wondered whether I could alleviate his condition.

TREATMENT

I mixed 2 per cent calendula and 2 per cent St John's Wort into a cream base containing *Lavandula cfficinalis* (lavender) for Charles to apply to his face and to his legs. I also gave him a 10 ml bottle of essential oils made up of *Mentha x piperita* (peppermint) and *Eucalyptus radiata* (eucalyptus) in equal proportions. He was to take 6 drops in a steam inhalation every morning.

I recommended that he should take 1,000 mg of vitamin C morning and evening and increase this dosage and the number of daily inhalations at the first sign of a cold.

OUTCOME

Charles appears for check-up appointments and repeat prescriptions. His face is rarely red now, the skin on his legs is no longer hard and bruised and there are no new varicose veins.

CASE SIX - LIZ

BACKGROUND

Liz, a 34-year-old woman I was helping through her first pregnancy, fell downstairs when she was twenty-nine weeks pregnant. She cracked one rib and was covered in bruises.

TREATMENT

After hospital treatment, I gave Liz pure arnica oil for her partner to massage gently around her rib area. In addition, I advised soaking in baths containing 6 drops of *Lauandula officinalis* (lavender) twice a day.

OUTCOME

After one week of the massage treatment, the pain in Liz's cracked rib had lessened and the bruising and stiffness were considerably reduced.

CASE SEVEN - HELEN

BACKGROUND

Helen, a sixty-year-old woman who ran a boarding kennels for dogs, was finding that when she got up in the mornings she could hardly move her fingers and wrists because they had so stiffened in the night.

TREATMENT

I mixed 2 per cent St John's wort with 2 per cent meadowsweet in a gel containing 3 per cent *Zingiber officinale* (ginger) and 1 per cent *Piper nigrum* (black pepper). I explained that I had calculated the preparation as well as I could with only these few personal details to guide me, and explained that she should apply the gel to her hands morning and night.

OUTCOME

After one month she ordered another jar and said her hands were pain free and had regained full mobility in the finger joints.

(For cases Five, Six and Seven, see Chapter Eight for information about combining macerated oils with essential oils.)

CASE EIGHT - JANET

BACKGROUND

When Janet, aged thirty-six, came to me in January 2012 she had just finished her fifth course of antibiotics taken within the last twelve months for a chronic urinary-tract infection. For the past five years she had suffered from persistent urethritis, involving an urgent and frequent desire to empty the bladder accompanied by general inflammation and discomfort in the vagina. Janet had stopped taking oral contraception six months ago and wanted to try for children but sexual intercourse with her partner was too painful.

A recent urine sample taken following the last antibiotic treatment was sent for microbiological investigation and proved to be 'sterile'. In other words it did not contain the level of pathogenic bacteria per millilitre of urine required by orthodox medicine to confirm a urinary tract infection. Yet Janet was in perpetual misery from her symptoms.

TREATMENT

I sent a vaginal swab and further urine samples to a laboratory for microscopy and culture. I then planned my selection of essential oils for treatment according to the findings that the bacteria *Escherichia coli* and *Klebsiella aerogenes* were present in the urino-genital area. The oils known to be active against these bacteria are *Cinnamomum zeylanicum* (cinnamon bark), *Melaleuca leucadendron*

(cajuput) and *Thymus vulgaris* thymol (red thyme). I then double-checked the validity of my stock of these oils with an aromatogram, and introduced them in turn to the

culture grown in the laboratory.

I included *Melaleuca alternifolia* (tea tree) because the long-term use of broad-spectrum antibiotics had also caused a candidiasis infection, popularly known as vaginal thrush, with the yeast-like fungus *Candida albicans.*

These 4 oils were mixed in equal proportions in a 50 per cent dilution with sunflower oil and applied 3 times a week in a is-minute abdominal and lower-back massage.

For home use I mixed a 3 per cent dilution of *Zingiber cifficinale* (ginger) and *Mentha x piperita* (peppermint) in equal proportions in sunflower oil to help with the constipation and the pain and inflammation respectively.

This was to be applied to the abdominal area once a day. I advised the nightly insertion of tampons soaked in 10 ml live yoghurt containing 10 drops of *Melaleuca alternifolia* to combat further the thrush.

Dietary changes were necessary too - vital for the successful treatment of thrush. The exclusion of sugars, fermented foods, alcohol and other aggravates was introduced slowly over the next four weeks. In addition I recommended a high fluid intake to flush out the bladder and to relieve the constipation. Janet took 6 acidophilus tablets a day in order to replenish the intestinal flora that would have been adversely affected by the courses of antibiotics she had taken.

OUTCOME

By the end of the month there was no vaginal discharge, itching, pain or inflammation. Janet said she felt revitalised and free from the permanent tiredness that had blighted everything. For the following six months the above treatment was repeated for the three days before menstruation because the symptoms would recur to a moderate degree at this time. In September of that year Janet conceived and now has a healthy son.

(See Chapter Ten for the discussion about how aromatology can be complementary to orthodox medical care.)

CASE NINE - DOMINIC

BACKGROUND

Dominic, a 41-year-old financial trader who worked long days at his desk in a City bank, sought my help in 2013 because he was feeling generally unwell and fatigued.

I took some preliminary information about his height, weight and previous medical history. He was over six feet tall and slightly overweight; he enjoyed daily business lunches with alcohol and had a glass of whisky every evening. Although he tried to get to the gym three times a week, his life was otherwise sedentary.

In 2012, following five years of chronic cholecystitis (inflammation of the gall bladder), his gall bladder was removed. He still suffered from intermittent colicky abdominal pain, similar to what he had experienced before the surgery, but diarrhoea was a new, additional symptom.

He complained of a tight feeling across the site of the operation. Upon examination I found the scar tissue was hard, prominent and irregular and that his abdomen was bloated.

In the last year Dominic had had frequent severe headaches for the first time in his life. He complained of stiffness in his neck and shoulders. He was tall and was often bent over his desk. It turned out, too, that he frequently hooked his telephone between his chin and his shoulder while keying into his computer. I recommended the use of telephone headsets and a course in Alexander technique to make him aware of his posture.

I suspected the headaches and the abdominal discomfort were connected and related to the history of large gallstones, a problem which had been relieved but not solved by the removal of his gall bladder. He had continued with a high-fat, high-protein diet, accompanied by high alcohol consumption. I advised dietary changes to a low-fat, high-fibre diet without caffeine or alcohol. I suggested that we might experiment with the type and amount of fibre he introduced into his meals, because symptoms of irritable bowel syndrome can get worse before they adapt and improve with such changes.

TREATMENT

Treatment consisted of massage sessions once a week using slightly sedative oils to settle the digestive system and relax the muscles. The mixtures of oil were 10 per cent dilutions in saillower and rose hip oils of any 4 of the following: *Lavandula angustifolia* (lavender), *Achillea millefolium* (yarrow), *Matricaria chamomilla* (German chamomile), *Citrus limon* (lemon), *Mentha x piperita* (peppermint) and *Citrus aurantium* var. *amara* (orange bigarade).

OUTCOME

After six weeks Dominic reported only back pain. He had considerably changed his diet and felt that he had renewed energy. We decided to continue with body massage to relax and loosen his muscles in conjunction with more regular work-ours involving stretch exercise and aerobic activity to achieve a weight loss and greater mobility.

(See Chapter Eleven for the description of the holistic approach of aromatologists.)

www.ingramcontent.com/pod-product-compliance
Lightning Source LLC
Chambersburg PA
CBHW071049290526
45795CB00004B/1406